*Lippincott's*
*Review Series*

# Maternal-Newborn Nursing

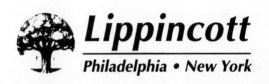

**Lippincott**

*Philadelphia • New York*

# *Lippincott's Review Series*

## SECOND EDITION

# *Maternal-Newborn Nursing*

**Barbara R. Stright,** RN, PhD
Associate Professor, School of Nursing
Clarion University of Pennsylvania
Clarion, Pennsylvania

**Lee-Olive Harrison,** RN, MEd
Associate Professor, School of Nursing
Clarion University of Pennsylvania
Clarion, Pennsylvania

*Acquisitions Editor:* **Susan Glover, RN, MSN**
*Sponsoring Editor:* **Deedie McMahon**
*Project Editor:* **Susan Deitch**
*Production Manager:* **Helen Ewan**
*Design Coordinator:* **Doug Smock**
*Indexer:* **Alexandra Nickerson**

RG951
.L57
1996

2nd Edition

**Library of Congress Cataloging in Publications Data**

Stright, Barbara R.
    Maternal-newborn nursing / Barbara R. Stright, Lee-Olive Harrison.
—2nd ed.
      p.   cm. — (Lippincott's review series)
    Earlier ed. was entered under the title.
    Includes bibliographical references and index.
    ISBN 0–397–55214–9
    1. Maternity nursing—Examinations, questions, etc.  2. Maternity
nursing—Outlines, syllabi, etc.  I. Harrison, Lee-Olive.
II. Title.  III. Series.
    [DNLM:  1. Maternal-Child Nursing—outlines.  2. Maternal-Child
Nursing—examination questions.  WY 18.2 S916m 1996]
    RG951.L57 1996
    610.73′678′076—dc20
    DNLM/DLC
    for Library of Congress                  95–25938
                                          CIP

9 8 7 6 5 4 3 2 1

To honor Barbara R. Stright, the best friend I could ever have.
I value and admire my partner, friend, confidant, confrere, and
colleague. It is her unselfishness and inspiration that made this book a reality.
**L.O.H.**


I attribute this work to those who touch my life, encourage me to dream,
wait with patience, and teach me with love and understanding.
**B.R.S.**

# REVIEWERS

---

**Lynne Hutnik Conrad, RN,C, MSN**
*Perinatal Clinical Nurse Specialist*
*Albert Einstein Medical Center*
*Philadelphia, Pennsylvania*

**Cecelia Tiller, RN, DSN**
*Assistant Professor*
*Medical College of Georgia School of Nursing*
*Augusta, Georgia*

# INTRODUCTION

Lippincott's Review Series is designed to help you in your study of the key subject areas in nursing. The series consists of six books, one in each core nursing subject area:

*Medical-Surgical Nursing*      *Mental Health and Psychiatric Nursing*
*Pediatric Nursing*             *Pathophysiology*
*Maternal-Newborn Nursing*      *Fluids and Electrolytes*

Each book contains a comprehensive outline content review, chapter study questions and answer keys with rationales for correct and incorrect responses, and a comprehensive examination and answer key with rationales for correct and incorrect responses.

Lippincott's Review Series was planned and developed in response to your requests for outline review books that address each major subject area and also contain a self-test mechanism. These books meet the need for comprehensive subject review books that will also assist you in identifying your strong and weak areas of knowledge. Each book is a complete source for review and self-assessment of a single core subject—all six together provide an excellent comprehensive review of entry-level nursing.

Each book is all-inclusive of the content addressed in major textbooks. The content outline review uses a consistent nursing process format throughout and addresses nursing care for well and ill clients. Also included are necessary teaching and other concepts, including growth and development, nutrition, pharmacology, and body structures, functions, and pathophysiology. Special features of each book are Key Concepts and Nursing Alerts, which are identified by distinctive icons. Key Concepts ☀ are basic facts the nurse needs to know to perform her job with ease and efficiency. Nursing Alerts ⚕ are fundamental guidelines the nurse can follow to ensure safe and effective care.

You can use the books in this series in several different ways. Overall, you can use them as subject reviews to augment general study throughout your basic nursing program and as a review to prepare for the National Council Licensure Examination (NCLEX-RN). How you use each book depends on your individual needs and preferences, and on whether you review each chapter systematically or concentrate only on those chapters whose subject areas are particularly problematic or challenging. You may instead choose to use the comprehensive examination as a self-assessment opportunity to evaluate your knowledge base before you review the content outline.

Likewise, you can use the study questions for pre- or post-testing after study, followed by the comprehensive examination as a means of evaluating your knowledge and competencies of an entire subject area.

Regardless of how you use the books, one of the strengths of the series is the self-assessment opportunity it offers in addition to guidance in studying and reviewing content. The chapter study questions and comprehensive examination questions have been carefully developed to cover all topics in the outline review. Most importantly, each question is categorized according to the components of the National Council of State Boards of Nursing Licensing Examination (NCLEX).

▶ Cognitive Level: Knowledge, Comprehension, Application, or Analysis
▶ Client Need: Safe, Effective Care Environment (Safe Care); Physiological Integrity (Physiologic); Psychosocial Integrity (Psychosocial); and Health Promotion and Maintenance (Health Promotion)
▶ Phase of the Nursing Process: Assessment, Analysis (Dx), Planning, Implementation, Evaluation

For those questions not related to a client need or to a phase of the nursing process, NA (not applicable) will be used, as in questions that test knowledge of a basic science.

Unlike the NCLEX examination that tests the cumulative knowledge needed for safe practice by an entry-level nurse, these practice tests systematically evaluate the knowledge base that serves as the building block for the entire nursing educational process. In this way, you can prepare for the NCLEX examination throughout your course of study. Good study habits throughout your educational program are not only the best way to ensure ongoing success, but also will prove the most beneficial way to prepare for the licensing examination.

Keep in mind that these books are not intended to replace formal learning. They cannot substitute for textbook reading, discussion with instructors, or class attendance. Every effort has been made to provide accurate and current information, but class attendance and interaction with an instructor will provide invaluable information not found in books. Used correctly, these books will help you increase understanding, improve comprehension, evaluate strengths and weaknesses in areas of knowledge, increase productive study time, and, as a result, help you improve your grades.

**MONEY BACK GUARANTEE**—Lippincott's Review Series will help you study more effectively during coursework throughout your educational program, and help you prepare for quizzes and tests, including the NCLEX exam. If you buy and use any of the six volumes in Lippincott's Review Series and fail the NCLEX exam, simply send us verification of your exam results and your copy of the review book to the address below. We will promptly send you a check for our suggested list price.

*Lippincott's Review Series*
Marketing Department
Lippincott-Raven Publishers
227 East Washington Square
Philadelphia, PA 19106-3780

# ACKNOWLEDGMENTS

---

We would like to thank Donna L. Hilton and Susan M. Keneally for working so closely with us to make this part of the *Lippincott's Review Series, Maternal-Newborn Nursing,* a reality. This was another challenge for us. We believe nursing students will also be challenged by using this series to increase their knowledge and comprehension of maternal-newborn care.

*The authors*

# CONTENTS

————————

*xiv*

# Lippincott's Review Series

# Maternal-Newborn Nursing

# Introduction to Maternal-Newborn Nursing

## I.  Evolution of maternal-newborn nursing

### A.  History of maternal-newborn care in America

1.  1700 to 1900

    a.  During this period, traditional English birth practices prevailed; improved maternal outcome in the colonies compared with Europe is attributed to less crowded conditions, better nutrition, and healthier women.

    b.  **Throughout history, midwives commonly attended births; formal training and licensure for physicians did not occur until the mid-19th century.**

    c.  Thereafter, for a short while, midwives and physicians commonly copracticed, with midwives being called for uncomplicated births and physicians attending complicated deliveries.

      d.    Analgesia for childbirth, introduced by Simpson in 1847, shifted childbirth from the home to the hospital by the early 20th century.

      e.    By the late 19th century, midwifery was fully absorbed into medical training as a specialty.

**2.** Early 20th century

      a.    **Before 1900, less than 5% of births in the United States occurred in hospitals. As medicine became more organized, hospitals opened in large numbers, providing a centralized setting for physician practice.**

      b.    The childbirth experience became dictated by strict hospital rules, separation of women from families during labor and birth, restriction of maternal activity during labor, transfer to delivery room for birth, and early transfer of newborn to nursery with no provisions for parent–newborn contact.

      c.    Hospitals developed training programs for nurses. Nursing students provided nursing care for hospitalized clients, and graduate nurses provided in-home nursing care as employees of the families.

      d.    Legislation was passed in many states outlawing midwifery practice because of the belief that hospital-based physician care was superior.

      e.    In 1918, the Maternity Center Association was founded in New York to provide care to poor women and children.

      f.    In 1925, the Frontier Nursing Service was established by Mary Breckinridge to provide care for families in remote areas of Appalachia.

**3.** Late 20th century

      a.    **In the late 1950s, a coalition of consumers, healthcare professionals, and childbirth educators began challenging the routine use of analgesics and anesthestics for childbirth. Standard obstetric practices for healthy women and newborns were challenged, as was exclusion of fathers from labor and birth. By the early 1970s, prepared childbirth, largely attributed to French obstetrician Fernand Lamaze, was a relatively common practice in the United States.**

      b.    Since the 1960s, two new medical specialties, perinatology and neonatology, have greatly affected the organization and delivery of perinatal care.

      c.    In 1969, the Nurses' Association of the American College of Obstetricians and Gynecologists (NAACOG) was formed. In 1992, this organization changed its name to the Association of Women's Health, Obstetric, and Neonatal Nurses (AWHONN).

    d.    By the 1970s, more than 90% of births in the United States were attended by physicians and occurred in hospitals. Since the 1970s, many restrictions on the location and scope of midwife practice have been rescinded, and by 1981, the services of a certified nurse midwife were reimbursable through Medicaid.

    e.    In 1986, the Division of Maternal-Child Nursing within the American Nurses Association was established.

  **4.**    20th-century nursing specialization

    a.    Just as healthcare in general and maternal-newborn care in particular have evolved, so has nursing care. Certified nurse-midwives, nurse practitioners, and clinical nurse specialists are key examples of expanded roles.

    b.    **Certified nurse-midwives**

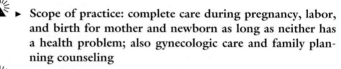

    ▶ **Scope of practice: complete care during pregnancy, labor, and birth for mother and newborn as long as neither has a health problem; also gynecologic care and family planning counseling**

    ▶ **Qualifications: RN; extensive study program combined with supervised clinical experience; testing and certification by the American College of Nurse-Midwives**

    c.    Nurse practitioners

        ▶ Scope of practice: primary care for specific groups of clients in collaboration with a physician for treatments and medications outside of the practitioner's scope of practice; specific client groups served by maternity nurse practitioners, family nurse practitioners, pediatric nurse practitioners, and family planning nurse practitioners

        ▶ Qualifications: RN; completion of accredited nurse practitioner program (such as the first nurse practitioner program begun at Massachusetts General Hospital in 1961)

    d.    Clinical nurse specialists

        ▶ Scope of practice: interventions in various problems encountered in maternal-newborn care; direct service to clients within the specialty field (eg, neonatology, pediatrics, neurology, gerontology); consultation services to other nurses; staff education programs and instruction in schools of nursing

        ▶ Qualifications: RN; master's degree

**B.**  **Influence of federal and state programs on maternal-newborn care**

  **1.**    In 1921, the Sheppard-Towner Act provided funds for state-managed maternal-child health programs.

  **2.**    In 1930, the Sheppard-Towner Act was repealed due to political pressure exerted by organized medicine, despite evidence that mortality rates declined under these programs.

3. In 1935, the Social Security Act was passed. Title V of the Act provides funding for maternal-child health programs.

4. In 1944, the Public Health Service Act provided funding for research and education of personnel needed for maternal and child health programs.

5. In 1962, the National Institute of Child Health and Human Development was authorized. The Institute supports research and training in special health problems and needs of mothers and children and funds basic science research relating to human growth and development, including prenatal development.

6. In 1964, the Title V amendment to the Public Health Service Act established the Maternal and Infant Care (MIC) projects, emphasizing comprehensive prenatal and newborn care in public centers.

7. In 1965, Title XIX of the Medicaid Program provided funds to facilitate care for pregnant women and young children.

 8. **In 1965, phenylketonuria testing became mandatory for all newborns in Illinois and Michigan, setting a precedent for other states.**

9. In 1966, the Department of Health, Education, and Welfare (HEW), which is now known as the Department of Health and Human Services (HHS), issued a policy statement on birth control, stating that the Department would support, on request, health programs making family planning information and services available.

10. In 1967, many states' Medicaid programs expanded to include care during pregnancy and child care.

11. In 1968, Head Start programs began providing educational opportunities for low-income preschool children.

12. In 1969, the National Center for Family Planning was established under the Health Services and Mental Health Administration, HEW, to serve as a clearing house for contraceptive information.

13. In 1973, the National Center on Child Abuse and Neglect was established in HEW's Office of Child Development to act as a clearing house for information about child abuse.

 14. **In 1975, the Women, Infants, and Children (WIC) program, a supplemental food program directed at providing supplemental food and nutrition education for low-income families, was established.**

15. In 1976, the Early and Periodic Screening, Diagnostic and Treatment (EPSDT) program began providing Medicaid-

eligible children with regular health screening and treatment through federal funding.

16. In 1977, the Child Health Assessment Act (CHAP) extended the EPSDT program to broaden eligibility and to require that treatment be given for conditions discovered during assessment.

17. In 1987, controlling healthcare costs became a major focus of the federal government and insurance companies. One major cost-controlling effort is prospective payment, in which payers (federal sources and insurance companies) agree in advance on a certain level of reimbursement for a particular kind of care, regardless of actual cost. This strategy was originally designed for Medicare. The level of reimbursement is determined by diagnosis-related groups.

**C. Development of nurse-midwifery in the United States**

1. In 1932, the Maternity Center Association began training public health nurses in midwifery practice in the Lobenstein School of Nurse-Midwifery. Elsewhere in the 1930s, the Frontier Nursing Service in Kentucky began training nurses in midwifery.

2. In 1969, the American College of Nurse-Midwives was established as the official agency for approving educational programs and certifying graduates of these programs.

3. In 1971, the first National Certification Examination for nurse-midwives was administered; the designation CNM indicates certified nurse-midwife.

4. In 1981, Congress authorized Medicaid payments for the services of certified nurse-midwives.

## II. Family-centered maternal-newborn nursing

**A. Description: Safe, quality nursing care that recognizes, focuses on, and adapts to the physical and psychosocial needs of the pregnant woman, family, and newborn. Family-centered nursing care fosters family unity and promotes and protects the physiologic well-being of the mother and child.**

**B. Development**

1. During the early 1940s, more parents began questioning the rigid hospital rules and routines associated with labor and delivery.

2. During this period, Grantly Dick-Reed introduced the concept of childbirth preparation and participation of the father in labor and delivery.

3. John Bowlby studied the effects of attachment (bonding), separation, and deprivation between mother and newborn.

4. Klaus and Kennell described the effects of maternal deprivation on children and did extensive studies on bonding.

    **5.** St. Mary's Hospital in Evansville, Indiana, established the first Family-Centered Maternity Care Program in the late 1950s; this approach quickly spread across the nation.

**C. Philosophy and features**

    **1.** The basic philosophy of family-centered maternal-newborn nursing can be summed up in the following statements:

        a. Given adequate information and professional support, the family is capable of making decisions about care during the childbearing periods.

        b. In most cases, childbirth is a normal, healthy event in the life of a family.

        c. Childbirth marks the beginning of a new set of important family relationships.

 **2. Important features of family-centered maternal-newborn care include:**

        a. **Prenatal and parent education classes**

        b. **Family participation in labor, birth, and the postpartum period, including attendance by the father or a support person during labor and birth, unrestricted family visitation, and sibling participation**

        c. **Presence of support person for complicated or cesarean birth, if possible**

        d. **Use of a homelike birth setting**

        e. **Flexible policies regarding routine procedures**

        f. **Postbirth recovery without routine transfer of family**

        g. **Early extended parent–newborn contact**

        h. **Flexible rooming-in policy**

        i. **Family involvement in special neonatal care unit, including transport of mother and newborn, if necessary**

        j. **Early postbirth discharge with close follow-up**

    **3.** Other aspects of family-centered maternal-newborn care may include:

        a. Nontraditional labor and birth settings (eg, in-hospital birth centers, freestanding birth centers, home birth)

        b. Nonviolent or gentle birth practices

        c. Single-room maternity systems, called labor, delivery, and recovery rooms or labor, delivery, recovery, postpartum rooms

## III. Ethical and legal issues in maternal-newborn care

   **A.** Complex ethical questions

      1. Maternal versus fetal rights

         a. Concept of the fetus as a client separate from the mother

         b. Possibility of forced medical treatment of the fetus against the wishes of the mother when fetal life and well-being do not exist independently of the mother and when the mother is required to undergo treatment against her will

      2. Widely varying standards of fetal viability

      3. Selective terminations of pregnancy

      4. Life support or withdrawal of life support in a critically ill newborn

      5. Human immunodeficiency virus testing of all pregnant women

   **B.** Litigation and professional liability

      1. Critical elements of professional practice in maternity nursing include:

         a. Thorough initial health history and physical examination, enabling the nurse to identify risk factors and institute appropriate measures

         b. Complete and accurate documentation of client status and care rendered, regarded as the only valid record of events from a legal standpoint

         c. Appropriate use and interpretation of fetal monitoring

      2. Nurses' and physicians' exposure to litigation in obstetric care is increasing. (Approximately 80% of all medical malpractice cases in U.S. history have been filed since 1975; nearly 75% of all obstetric or gynecologic physicians in the United States have been sued, and 30% of these have had three or more suits filed against them.)

      3. Joint actions against the physician and nurse are common, especially in emergency situations in which assessments and interventions occur quickly.

      **4. Most of the increased litigation results from allegations related to severe newborn birth injuries:**

         a. **Caused by substandard care and requiring long-term therapy**

         b. **Resulting from unavailability of physician**

      5. With increased litigation comes increased liability insurance rates for nurses and physicians caring for childbearing families.

## IV. Implications for nursing management

### A. Assessment

1. Nursing assessment of the client and family includes:
   a. Nursing health history
   b. Interview and observation
   c. Measurement of vital signs and physiologic indicators
   d. Review of medical records
2. Various standardized tools (Table 1-1) can aid assessment.

### B. Nursing diagnoses

1. North American Nursing Diagnosis Association (NANDA) nursing diagnosis categories that typically apply to parents or other family members:
   a. Anxiety
   b. Constipation
   c. Ineffective Breastfeeding
   d. Family Coping: Potential for Growth
   e. Ineffective Family Coping: Compromised
   f. Decisional Conflict
   g. Fatigue
   h. Fear
   i. Anticipatory Grieving
   j. Dysfunctional Grieving
   k. Altered Health Maintenance
   l. Risk for Infection
   m. Knowledge Deficit
   n. Altered Nutrition: Less than body requirements
   o. Altered Nutrition: More than body requirements
   p. Pain
   q. Altered Parenting
   r. Self Esteem Disturbance
   s. Altered Patterns of Sexuality
   t. Altered Patterns of Urinary Elimination
2. NANDA nursing diagnoses that typically apply to the newborn:
   a. Risk for Altered Body Temperature
   b. Ineffective Breathing Pattern
   c. Diarrhea
   d. Risk for Infection
   e. Altered Nutrition: Less than body requirements
   f. Altered Nutrition: More than body requirements
   g. Pain
   h. Impaired Tissue Integrity

### C. Planning and implementation

1. Nursing intervention in maternal-newborn care involves activities designed to promote positive adaptation and high-level

TABLE 1-1.
Assessment Tools Used in Maternal-Newborn Nursing

| TOOL | PURPOSE | DESCRIPTION |
|---|---|---|
| Maternal-Fetal Attachment Scale (parent self-report) | ▶ Measures aspects of maternal attachment to fetus (A paternal version has been developed and tested.) | This contains 33 scales focusing on differentiation of self from fetus, interaction with fetus, attribution of characteristics to fetus, giving of self, and role taking. |
| Apgar scoring system | ▶ Allows quick, comprehensive evaluation of newborn's immediate adaptation to birth process and extrauterine life<br>▶ Indicates extent to which newborn requires more vigorous management or resuscitation | This rates five components (heart rate, respiratory effort, muscle tone, reflex irritability, and color), each on a scale from 0 to 2. Ratings are done at 1 and 5 minutes after birth. Scores of 0 to 3 reflect severe distress; 4 to 6, moderate distress; and 7 to 10, mild or absent distress. If the score is less than 6 at 5 min, assessment should be repeated at 10 min. |
| Brazelton Neonatal Behavior Assessment Scale (completed by professional) | ▶ Assesses social and interactive behavior of newborns from birth to 1 mo<br>▶ May be used to examine early individual differences in newborns<br>▶ Has been used in nursing as a strategy for teaching parents about newborn capabilities | Examination guide contains 27 reflex items, 27 behavioral reponse items, and ratings of newborn's predominant states, need for stimulation, and self-quieting activities. Typical examination requires 30 minutes. Training is necessary to establish skill in evolution. |
| Neonatal Perception Inventories (parent self-report) | ▶ Measures maternal perception of newborn, comparing a hypothetical "average" newborn with perception of own newborn. Based on the assumption that a mother ideally will rate her own newborn better than average | Scale asks for rating of own newborn and average newborn on six characteristics; sleeping, feeding, spitting up, elimination, crying, and predictability of behavior. Useful in combination, with other assessments of maternal–newborn relationships. |
| Home Observation Measurement of Environment (birth to 3 years; completed by professional) | ▶ Identifies aspects of environment that enhance newborn development | Comprises observation of 1 h in home on six subscales focusing on maternal responsiveness and organization of physical (especially play) environment. |

*Source: May, K. A., & Mahlmeister, L. R. (1994). Maternal and neonatal nursing: Family-centered care (3rd ed.). Philadelphia: J.B. Lippincott.*

wellness. Interventions encompass everything from comfort measures to counseling and health education.

2. Dissemination of the plan for care to others responsible for providing care is essential to provide continuity and safety.

3. Specific client problems, expected outcomes, and appropriate interventions for each problem need to be documented.

4. Client teaching for self-care is a primary nursing intervention with healthy childbearing families and is based on such considerations as:
   a. Client or family learning needs
   b. Principles of teaching and learning
   c. Physical and psychological condition of client and family
   d. Sociocultural factors

**D. Evaluation**

1. Appropriate evaluation involves:
   a. Establishing criteria for observation and measurement
   b. Assessing current responses for evidence of progress
   c. Comparing current responses to the established criteria
2. Any statement of the effectiveness and reliability of nursing actions is best made with qualifications indicating the degree or amount of effectiveness and the reliability claimed.
3. Nursing evaluation of actual outcomes may then lead to a reassessment and adjustment in the plan of care or refocusing on other identified problems.

## Bibliography

Bobak, I. M., & Jensen, M. D. (1993). *Maternity and gynecologic care: The nurse and the family* (5th ed.). St Louis: C.V. Mosby.

May, K. A., & Mahlmeister, L. R. (1994). *Maternal and neonatal nursing: Family-centered care* (3rd ed.). Philadelphia: J.B. Lippincott.

Reeder, S. J., Martin, L. L., & Koniak, D. (1992). *Maternity nursing: Family, newborn, and women's health care* (17th ed.). Philadelphia: J.B. Lippincott.

# STUDY QUESTIONS

1. Title V of the Social Security Act accomplished which of the following?
   a. Nurse-midwifery in the United States
   b. First federal involvement in maternity care
   c. Comprehensive prenatal and newborn care in public clinics
   d. Federal funding for maternal-child health care

2. Which of the following would be considered a feature of traditional rather than comprehensive family-centered birth care?
   a. Transfer from labor room to delivery room
   b. Prenatal and parent education opportunities
   c. Accommodation for presence of support person at a cesarean birth
   d. Early postbirth discharge and planned follow-up care

3. Once a mother has given birth, which assessment tool would the nurse be most likely to use to determine the newborn's initial adjustment to the extrauterine environment?
   a. Apgar Scoring System
   b. Home Observation Measurement of Environment (HOME)
   c. Brazelton Neonatal Behavior Assessment Scale (BNBAS)
   d. Neonatal Perception Inventories (NPI)

4. In which century did a majority of babies begin to be born in hospitals?
   a. 17th
   b. 18th
   c. 19th
   d. 20th

5. An important federal program that provides supplemental food to low-income families is known by which of the following acronyms?
   a. CHAP
   b. EPSDT
   c. WIC
   d. CNM

6. Which of the following is most typical of traditional care in maternity nursing?
   a. Homelike atmosphere for birth
   b. Early parent–newborn contact
   c. Scheduled newborn feedings
   d. Father participating as coach

7. In maternal-child care, the most commonly filed lawsuit involves which of the following claims?
   a. Birth injury to the newborn related to substandard care
   b. Maternal injury as a result of cesarean section birth
   c. Maternal death resulting from physician error
   d. Newborn death resulting from physician incompetence

8. Which agency was founded in 1962 to support research and training related to prenatal development?
   a. The National Center for Family Planning
   b. The National Institute of Child Health and Human Development
   c. The Department of Health, Education, and Welfare
   d. The National Commission of Nursing Implementation Project

9. The first organized midwifery service in the United States was founded in 1925 by:
   a. Lillian D. Wald
   b. Lavinia L. Dock
   c. Isabel H. Robb
   d. Mary Breckinridge

10. Natural, or prepared, childbirth practices are primarily associated with:
    a. Leboyer
    b. Lemaze
    c. Bowlby
    d. Dick-Reed

# ANSWER KEY

1. **Correct response: d**
   The 1935 Amendment to Title V provided federal funding for maternal-child health care.
   a. Organized nurse-midwifery grew out of the activities of the Maternity Center Association in New York City.
   b. The Sheppard-Towner Act of 1921 marked the first federal involvement in maternity care.
   c. The MIC projects emphasized comprehensive prenatal and newborn care in public clinics.
   *Knowledge/Health Promotion/NA*

2. **Correct response: a**
   Transfer from labor room to delivery room is a characteristic of traditional care.
   b, c, and d. These are all characteristics of family-centered care.
   *Knowledge/Health Promotion/NA*

3. **Correct response: a**
   The Apgar score measures the newborn's immediate adjustment to life after 1 minute and again after 5 minutes. Assessment components include heart rate, respiratory effort, muscle tone, reflexes, and color.
   b. HOME focuses on maternal responsiveness and the newborn's physical environment.
   c. BNBAS assesses the newborn's social behaviors from birth to 1 month.
   d. Completed by the parent, NPI measures the parent's perception of the newborn.
   *Physiologic/Knowledge/Assessment*

4. **Correct response: d**
   Most births did not occur in hospitals until the 1900s.
   a, b, and c. These timeframes are all too early.
   *Knowledge/Health Promotion/NA*

5. **Correct response: c**
   The WIC program deals with food and nutrition.
   a. CHAP refers to Child Health Assessment Act.
   b. EPSDT is the Early and Periodic Screening Diagnostic and Treatment Program.
   d. CNM stands for certified nurse-midwife.
   *Comprehension/Health Promotion/NA*

6. **Correct response: c**
   Rigid scheduling of newborn feeding and care routines are examples of traditional maternity nursing.
   a, b, and d. These aspects are more typical of family-centered birth care.
   *Comprehension/Health Promotion/Planning*

7. **Correct response: a**
   Birth injury with long-term consequences is the most frequently filed claim in obstetric law suits.
   b, c, and d. These claims are less common than birth injury.
   *Comprehensive/Safe Care/NA*

8. **Correct response: b**
   The National Institute of Child Health and Human Development was established in 1962 to support research involving prenatal development.
   a. The NCFP was established in 1969 under HEW to serve as a clearing house for contraceptive information.
   c. HEW, the forerunner of HHS, was established in 1953. It was responsible for programs in public health, education, and economic security.
   d. HHS was established in 1980 to protect and advance the health of the American people.
   *Knowledge/NA/NA*

9. **Correct response: d**
   Mary Breckinridge founded the Fron-

tier Nursing Service, the first organized midwifery service, in 1925.
a. Lillian Wald established the House on Henry Street and initiated public school nursing in 1902.
b. Lavinia Dock was a prominent suffragist and feminist.
c. Isabel Robb organized the Johns Hopkins Hospital School of Nursing and was founder of the American Journal of Nursing.
*Knowledge/NA/NA*

10. *Correct response: b*
Lamaze is generally associated with natural childbirth practices.
a. Dr. Frederick Leboyer, a French obstetrician, suggested new delivery room procedures to make birth less traumatic for the newborn.
c. John Bowlby described the impact of maternal separation on children.
d. Grantly Dick-Reed introduced the concept of prepared childbirth.
*Knowledge/NA/NA*

# Sexuality and Reproduction

## I.  Overview

### A.  Sexuality

1.  A person's sexuality encompasses complex emotions, attitudes, preferences, and behaviors related to expression of the sexual self and eroticism.

2.  Sexual relationships are a dynamic aspect of life, intertwined with biologic and psychosocial components.

3.  Nurses commonly are resource people for clients seeking information related to human sexuality and functioning during the reproductive years.

    **4.** Developmental tasks of sexual identity include:
- a. *Gender identity:* sense of masculinity and femininity; thought to be established in part by how the individual was treated by his or her parents as a child
- b. *Sex role standards:* behavior, attributes, and attitudes that differentiate roles
- c. *Sexual partner preference:* heterosexual, homosexual, or bisexual; may vary during lifetime; probably shaped by complex interaction of several factors, including prenatal hormone environment, early parent interactions, social mores and values, family dynamics, and imitation of most valued parent

    **5.** Responsible sexuality involves commitment to a relationship, responsible reproductive health care, and rational decisions about childbearing.

**B. Male and female reproductive potentials**

    **1.** A woman's reproductive lifespan is finite; it begins shortly after menarche (between 10 and 13 years), declines somewhat during the late reproductive years, and terminates with menopause. The average age of naturally occurring menopause is 51.4 years, with an age range of 35 to 60 years.

    **2.** The large initial store of germ cells (primordial ova) present at birth represents the total ova formed during the lifespan. By way of atresia, these germ cells decrease in number; by puberty, only 300,000 of the 6 to 7 million fetal germ cells remain. *A woman releases no more than 500 ova during ovulation throughout her lifetime.*

    **3.** A woman's capacity to reproduce may be disassociated from sexual excitement or receptivity.

    **4.** Reproductive activity in the male begins with sperm production at the onset of puberty and continues throughout his lifespan.

    **5.** New sperm cells are generated every 74 days. *Billions of mature sperm are produced during a man's normal lifespan.*

    **6.** A man's capacity to reproduce is associated with sexual excitement, penile erection, and ejaculation.

**II. Female reproductive system**

**A. External organs**

    **1.** Mons pubis: a mound of fatty tissue over the symphysis pubis that cushions and protects the bone

    **2.** Labia majora: longitudinal folds of pigmented skin extending from the mons pubis to the perineum

    **3.** Labia minora: soft longitudinal skin folds between the labia majora

4. Clitoris: erectile tissue located at the upper end of the labia minora; primary site of sexual arousal
5. Urethral meatus (urethral orifice): small opening of urethra located between clitoris and vaginal orifice for the purpose of urination
6. Skene's or paraurethral glands: small mucus-secreting glands that open into the posterior wall of the urinary meatus and lubricate the vagina
7. Vestibule: an almond-shaped area between the labia minora containing the vaginal introitus, hymen, and Bartholin's glands
8. Vaginal introitus: external opening of the vagina
9. Hymen: membranous tissue ringing the vaginal introitus
10. Bartholin's or vulvovaginal glands: mucus-secreting glands located on either side of the vaginal orifice
11. Perineal body; muscles and fascia that support pelvic structures

 12. **Perineum: tissue between the anus and vagina; the area where episiotomy is performed**

**B. Internal organs**

1. Vagina: the female organ of copulation; a tubular musculomembranous organ lying between the rectum and the urethra and bladder; also known as the birth canal (Fig. 2-1)
2. Uterus: a hollow, muscular organ with three muscle layers (perimetrium, myometrium, and endometrium) located between the bladder and rectum and consisting of the fundus, body (corpus), and cervix; uterine functions include:

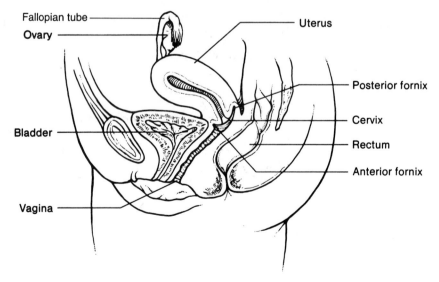

FIGURE 2-1.
Lateral cross-section of internal female reproductive structures.

a. Menstruation: sloughing away of spongy layers of endometrium with bleeding from torn vessels

b. Pregnancy: environment of developing embryo and fetus after fertilization

c. Labor: powerful contractions of muscular uterine wall that result in expulsion of fetus

3. Uterine ligaments include:

a. Broad and round ligaments, which provide upper support for the uterus

b. Cardinal, pubocervical, and uterosacral ligaments, which are suspensory and provide middle support

c. Pelvic muscular floor ligaments, which provide lower support

4. Fallopian tubes: tubes that extend from the upper outer angles of the uterus and end near the ovary; passageway for the ovum to travel from the ovary to the uterus and for the sperm to travel from the uterus to the ovary

5. Ovaries: female sex glands located on each side of the uterus with two functions:

a. Ovulation (release of ovum)

b. Secretion of hormones (estrogen and progesterone)

C. Pelvis

1. The pelvis is a bony ring in the lower portion of the trunk, consisting of three parts (ilium, ischium, and pubis) and four bones (two innominate bones or hipbones, sacrum, and coccyx).

2. The pelvic bones are held together by four joints (articulations): symphysis pubis, two sacroiliac, and sacrococcygeal. Fibrocartilage between these joints provides movability.

3. Types of pelves include:

a. Gynecoid: typical female pelvis with rounded inlet

b. Android: normal male pelvis with heart-shaped inlet

c. Anthropoid: "ape-like" pelvis with oval inlet

d. Platypelloid: flat, female-type pelvis with transverse oval inlet

4. Pelvic size and structural irregularities can alter labor and birth.

5. Pelvimetry (the process of measuring the internal or external pelvis) is performed with pelvimetery, radiography, or internal examination.

a. *Internal pelvic inlet measurement:* diagonal conjugate— lower margin of symphysis pubis to promontory of sacrum; normally 12.5 to 13 cm

b. *Internal midpelvic measurement:* distance between ischial spines and prominence or bluntness of spines; normally 10.5 cm

      c.   *Internal pelvic outlet measurement:* estimation of width of pubic arch, mobility of coccyx, intertuberous diameter, and posterior sagittal diameter

**D.   Breasts**

   **1.**   The female breasts (mammary glands) are specialized sebaceous glands that produce milk after childbirth (lactation).

   **2.**   Internal breast structures include:

      a.   Glandular tissue (parenchyma): acini (milk-producing cells), which cluster in groups of 15 to 20 to form the lobes of the breast

      b.   Lactiferous ducts or sinuses, which form passageways from the lobes to the nipple

      c.   Fibrous tissue: Cooper's ligaments, which provide support to the mammary glands

      d.   Adipose and fibrous tissue (stroma), which provides the relative size and consistency of the breast

   **3.**   External structures include:

      a.   Nipple: raised, pigmented area of the breast

      b.   Areola: pigmented skin around nipple

      c.   Montgomery's tubercles: sebaceous glands of the areola

   **4.**   The breasts change in size and nodularity in response to cyclic ovarian hormonal changes, including:

      a.   Estrogen stimulation, producing tenderness

      b.   Progesterone (postovulation), causing increased tenderness and breast enlargement

   **5.**   **Physical changes in breast size and activity are at a minimum 5 to 7 days after menstruation stops; this is the best time to detect pathologic changes through breast self-examination.**

**E.   Menstrual cycle and hormones**

   **1.**   The menstrual cycle is a monthly cyclical pattern of ovulation and menstruation, involving:

      a.   Ovulation: discharge of mature ovum from ovary

      b.   Menstruation: periodic shedding of blood and mucous epithelial cells from the uterus; average blood loss, 50 mL (¼ cup)

   **2.**   Menarche (onset of menstruation) typically occurs between 10 and 13 years.

   **3.**   The ovary produces mature gametes and secretes the following hormones:

      a.   Estrogen: contributes to characteristics of femaleness (eg, female body build, breast growth)

      b.   Progesterone (hormone of pregnancy): quiets or decreases contractility of the uterus

c.  Prostaglandins: regulate reproductive process (stimulate contractility of uterine and other smooth muscles)

**4. The menstrual cycle occurs in four levels: central nervous system (CNS; hypothalamic-pituitary), ovarian, endometrial (menstrual), and cervical levels.**

5.  At the CNS level:

a.  The hypothalamus stimulates the anterior pituitary gland by secreting gonadotropin-releasing hormone (GnRH). The anterior pituitary secretes two gonadotropins: follicle-stimulating hormone (FSH) and luteinizing hormone (LH).

b.  FSH prompts the ovary to develop ovarian follicles; the developing follicles secrete estrogen, which feeds back to the anterior pituitary to suppress FSH and trigger a surge of LH.

c.  LH acts with FSH to cause ovulation and enhance corpus luteum formation.

6.  At the ovarian level (two phases):

a.  An oocyte grows within the primordial follicle in two phases: follicular and luteal.

b.  In the follicular phase (days 1–14), the follicle matures due to FSH.

c.  In the luteal phase (days 15–22), the corpus luteum develops from a ruptured follicle.

7.  At the endometrial level (four phases):

a.  In the menstrual phase (days 1–5), the estrogen level is low, and cervical mucus is scanty.

b.  In the proliferative (follicular) phase (days 6–14), the estrogen level is high, the endometrium and myometrium thicken, and changes in cervical mucosa occur. (Note: Variations in the menstrual cycle are due to variations in the number of days in this phase.) On average, *ovulation occurs on day 14 of a 28-day cycle.*

c.  In the secretory phase (days 14–26), after release of the ovum, the estrogen level drops, progesterone level is high, increased uterine vascularity occurs, and tissue glycogen levels increase.

d.  In the ischemic phase (days 27–28), estrogen and progesterone levels recede, arterial vessels constrict, the endometrium prepares to shed, the blood vessels rupture, and menstruation begins.

8.  At the cervical level:

a.  Before ovulation, estrogen levels rise, causing cervical os dilation, abundant liquid mucus, high spinnbarkeit, and excellent sperm penetration.

       b.    Postovulation, progesterone levels rise, resulting in cervical os constriction, scant viscous mucus, low spinnbarkeit, no ferning, and poor sperm penetration.

       c.    During pregnancy, cervical circulation (blood supply) increases, and a protective mucus plug forms.

**F.   Climacteric**

    **1.**    The climacteric is a transitional period during which ovarian function and hormonal production decline.

    **2.**    **Menopause refers to a woman's last menstrual period; the average age of menopause is 51.4 years.**

    **3.**    Women may ovulate after menopause and thus can become pregnant.

# III.   Male reproductive system

  **A.**   **External structures**

      **1.**    Penis: the male organ of copulation (Fig. 2-2). This cylindrical shaft consisting of the following:

         a.    Two lateral columns of erectile tissue (corpora cavernosa)

         b.    A column of erectile tissue on the underside of the penis (corpus spongiosum) that encases the urethra

         c.    The glans penis, a cone-shaped expansion of the corpus spongiosum that is highly sensitive to sexual stimulus

         d.    The prepuce, or foreskin, a skin flap that covers the glans penis in uncircumcised males

      **2.**    Scrotum: a pouch hanging below the penis that contains the

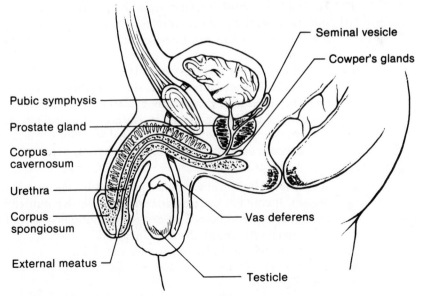

FIGURE 2-2.
Lateral cross-section of male reproductive structures.

testes. Internally, the medial septum divides the scrotum into two sacs, each of which contains a testis.

**B.** **Internal structures**

1. Testes: two solid ovoid organs 4 to 5 cm long, divided into lobes containing seminiferous tubules, where spermatogenesis occurs. Functions include production of testosterone and spermatogenesis.

2. Epididymis: a tubular sac located next to each testis that is a reservoir for sperm storage and maturation

3. Vas deferens: a duct extending from the epididymis to the ejaculatory duct, providing a passageway for sperm

4. Ejaculatory duct: the canal formed by the union of the vas deferens and the excretory duct of the seminal vesicle, which enters the urethra at the prostate gland

5. Urethra: the passageway for urine and semen, extending from the bladder to the urethral meatus

**C.** **Accessory glands**

1. Other structures in the male reproductive system produce secretions that facilitate transportation of spermatozoa along the urethra during ejaculation and provide a temporary safe milieu for the fragile sperm. The function of the accessory glands is maintained by testosterone.

2. Seminal vesicles that are located behind the bladder and in front of the rectum deliver secretions to the urethra through the ejaculatory ducts.

3. The prostate gland, which surrounds the base of the urethra and the ejaculatory duct, secretes a clear fluid with a slightly acid pH rich in acid phosphatase, citric acid, zinc, and proteolytic enzymes.

4. Bulbourethral and urethral glands (Cowper's glands) lie at the base of the prostate and on either side of the membranous urethra; they produce a clear, alkaline mucinous substance that lubricates the urethra and coats its surface. The alkalinity assists in neutralizing the acidic female vaginal secretions, which otherwise would be detrimental to sperm survival.

**D.** **Semen**

1. Semen is a thick, whitish fluid ejaculated by the man during orgasm. It contains spermatozoa and fructose-rich nutrients.

2. During ejaculation, semen receives contributions of fluid from the seminal vesicles and the prostate gland.

3. Combined semen is alkaline (average pH, 7.5).

4. The average amount of semen released during ejaculation is 2.5 to 3.5 mL.

**E.** **Male breasts**

    **1.** Male mammary tissue remains dormant throughout life, but the breasts are a site of sexual excitation and arousal.

    **2.** Although rare (accounting for less than 1% of all breast cancers in the United States), male breast cancer occurs frequently enough to warrant routine inspection of the breasts for dimpling, discharge, or nipple inversion.

**F.** **Neurohormonal control of the male reproductive system**

    **1.** At puberty, the hypothalamus stimulates the pituitary to produce FSH and LH.

    **2.** FSH stimulates germ cells within the testes to manufacture sperm.

    **3.** LH stimulates the production of testosterone in the testes.

    **4.** Testosterone, one of several androgens (and the most potent) produced in the testes, is responsible for the development of secondary sex characteristics at puberty.

    **5.** Testosterone production occurs in the interstitial Leydig cells in the seminiferous tubules. Leydig cells are abundant in the newborn and pubescent male, and testosterone is abundant during these periods. Testosterone production slows after 40 years; by 80 years, production is only about one-fifth peak level.

    **6.** Although LH stimulates the Leydig cells to produce testosterone from cholesterol, testosterone inhibits the secretion of LH by the anterior pituitary.

    **7.** Spermatogenesis (sperm production) occurs continually after puberty, providing large numbers of sperm for unlimited ejaculations during the mature lifespan.

    **8.** Spermatozoa are released from the epithelial wall of the seminiferous tubules. Meiosis occurs during the process, and the number of chromosomes in each cell is reduced by one-half (haploid number).

    **9.** Spermatogenesis is a heat-sensitive process; the 2° to 3°F difference between scrotal and abdominal temperatures allows spermatogenesis to proceed in the cooler environment.

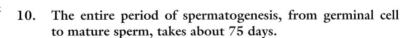     **10.** **The entire period of spermatogenesis, from germinal cell to mature sperm, takes about 75 days.**

**IV.** **Sexual response**

  **A.** **Female sexual response cycle**

    **1.** *Excitement phase*

      a. Vaginal lubrication occurs.

      b. The inner two-thirds of the vagina begins to lengthen and distend, and the outer one-third undergoes slight thickening.

    c.    The body of the uterus is pulled upward.

    d.    The vaginal walls become congested with blood and darken in color.

    e.    The clitoris increases in diameter, possibly with slightly increased tumescence of the glans clitoris.

    f.    The labia minora become engorged with blood and increase in size.

    g.    The labia majora flatten somewhat and retract away from the middle of the vulva.

    h.    The nipples become erect, and breast size increases.

    i.    Flushing occurs in approximately 75% of women.

    j.    Overall muscle tension increases.

2.  *Plateau phase*

    a.    The walls of the outer one-third of the vagina become further engorged with blood, decreasing the internal vaginal diameter.

    b.    The labia minora become further engorged with blood and darken and swell.

    c.    The clitoris retracts and is covered by the clitoral hood; the clitoral body decreases in size by about 50%.

    d.    The nipples become further engorged.

    e.    Flushing may spread to the abdomen, thighs, and back.

    f.    Muscle tension increases. Breathing becomes deeper; heart rate and blood pressure increase markedly as tension rises toward orgasm.

3.  *Orgasmic phase*

    a.    Strong muscular contractions occur in the outer one-third of the vagina, and the inner two-thirds expands.

    b.    The uterine muscles contract.

    c.    No observable changes occur in the labia majora, labia minora, clitoris, or breasts.

    d.    Flushing reaches a peak of color intensity and distribution.

    e.    Possibly strong muscular contractions, both voluntary and involuntary, may occur in many parts of the body, including the rectal sphincter muscle.

    f.    Respiratory rate may reach a peak of two to three times normal, heart rate may double, and blood pressure may increase as much as one-third above normal.

4.  *Resolution*

    a.    Blood engorging the walls of the outer one-third of the vagina disperses rapidly.

    b.    The inner two-thirds of the vagina gradually shrinks, and color returns to preexcitement shade.

    c.    The uterus descends, and the cervix dips into the seminal pool.

d.  The labia minora and majora return to unstimulated thickness and close toward midline.
e.  The clitoris protrudes from under the clitoral hood, and eventually returns to prestimulated size.
f.  Flushing disappears.
g.  Muscles relax quickly.
h.  Heart rate and blood pressure return to normal.

**B.  Male sexual response cycle**

1.  *Excitement phase*
    a.  Penile erection begins.
    b.  Scrotal skin becomes congested and thick.
    c.  Testes elevate into the scrotal sac.
    d.  Some nipple erection may occur.
    e.  Flushing may occur.
    f.  Heart rate and blood pressure begin to increase.
    g.  Generalized muscle tension increases, with a tendency toward involuntary muscle contractions.

2.  *Plateau phase*
    a.  The penis further enlarges, sometimes undergoing color changes corresponding to reddening of female labia.
    b.  Preorgasmic emission may occur from Cowper's glands.
    c.  The testes continue to be elevated, enlarge, and rotate (approximately 30 degrees).
    d.  Heart rate, blood pressure, and respiratory rate continue to increase.
    e.  Muscle tension increases.

3.  *Orgasmic phase*
     a.  **Rhythmic contractions expel semen from the epididymis through the vas deferens, seminal vesicles, prostate gland, urethra, and out the urethral meatus.**
    b.  Testes are at maximum elevation, size, and rotation.
    c.  Flushing reaches its peak.
    d.  Heart and respiratory rates also peak.
    e.  A general loss of voluntary control occurs.
    f.  A refractory period begins as the final contractions of the urethral walls occur.

4.  *Resolution phase*
    a.  More than 50% of the erection is lost rapidly in the first stage of resolution, with the penis gradually returning to its unstimulated size during the second stage.
    b.  The scrotum gradually loses its congested and thick status.
    c.  The testes descend and return to normal size.
    d.  Nipple erection subsides.
    e.  Flushing disappears.

f.   Heart rate, blood pressure, and respiratory rate return to normal.

g.   General muscle relaxation occurs.

**C.   Differences in male and female sexual response**

1.   **Women have three identifiable sexual response patterns:**

a.   Rapid progression to plateau stage with some peaks and valleys and one intense orgasm followed by rapid resolution; resembles the male pattern

b.   Steady progression to plateau stage followed by an intense orgasm and possibly subsequent orgasms, with slower resolution

c.   Slower progression to plateau stage followed by minor surges toward orgasm, causing prolonged pleasurable feelings without definitive orgasm

2.   **Men have one basic sexual response pattern:**

a.   Excitement progresses steadily to plateau stage, with one intense orgasm followed by resolution.

3.   In general, women experience orgasms in a wider range of duration and intensity than do men.

4.   Female orgasmic contractions last twice as long as the man's; the strength of the contractions is not as markedly concentrated in the first few pulsations.

**D.   Sexual concerns related to pregnancy**

1.   During pregnancy, the woman's desire for sex may be altered due to fatigue, nausea, and other discomforts of pregnancy.

2.   Other common sexual concerns during pregnancy include dyspareunia and male erectile dysfunction.

3.   Breasts may be painful to touch, especially during the first trimester.

4.   Some men may find the normal increase in the amount and odor of vaginal discharge during pregnancy a "turn off"; others do not.

5.   **Some women and couples need "permission" to be sexually active during pregnancy, along with reassurance that female orgasm will not harm the fetus.**

6.   For a couple who cannot have or who choose not to have intercourse during pregnancy, kissing, hugging, and oral or manual genital stimulation can be satisfying expressions of closeness and intimacy.

**V.   Implications for nursing management**

**A.   Assessment**

1.   Before interacting with any client regarding sexuality and reproduction, the nurse must perform a self-assessment; personal

attitudes and values will greatly influence the nursing care provided.

2.  A sexual history involves gathering information about the client or couple:
    a.  Past and current experiences with sexual activity
    b.  Sexual knowledge and how it was obtained
    c.  Attitudes toward sexuality
    d.  Current problem, if any

**B.  Nursing diagnoses**
1.  Anxiety
2.  Body Image Disturbance
3.  Ineffective Individual Coping
4.  Knowledge Deficit
5.  Self Esteem Disturbance
6.  Sexual Dysfunction
7.  Altered Sexuality Patterns

**C.  Planning and implementation**
1.  Create a private, trusting milieu to encourage clients to discuss sexual issues openly and to relieve anxiety.
2.  Validate and reassure clients about the universality of their sexual concerns.
3.  Provide information about alternate means of sexual expression, if appropriate.
4.  Refer clients with complex problems to professionals specializing in sexuality issues.

**D.  Evaluation**
1.  The client or couple verbalizes mutual satisfaction with choices regarding sexuality.
2.  The client or couple continues to make adjustments regarding sexuality throughout the pregnancy.

## Bibliography

Bobak, I. M., & Jensen, M. D. (1993). *Maternity and gynecologic care—the nurse and the family* (5th ed.). St. Louis: C.V. Mosby.

May, K. A., & Mahlmeister, L. R. (1994). *Maternal and neonatal nursing: Family-centered care* (3rd ed.). Philadelphia: J.B. Lippincott.

Reeder, S. J., Martin, L. L., & Koniak, D. (1992). *Maternity nursing: Family, newborn, and women's health care* (17th ed.). Philadelphia: J.B. Lippincott.

## STUDY QUESTIONS

28

1. Days 6 through 14 of the menstrual cycle constitute which of the following phases?
   a. Estrogen   *hormone*
   b. Proliferative   *is happens*
   c. Luteal   *in that one*
   d. Secretory

2. Which of the following reproductive organs contains the perimetrium, myometrium, and endometrium?
   a. Decidua
   b. Ovaries
   c. Uterus
   d. Vagina

3. The tissue between the vaginal orifice and the anus is known as the:
   a. mons pubis
   b. perineum
   c. hymen
   d. vestibule

4. Which breast structure is responsible for milk production?
   a. Acini cells
   b. Areola
   c. Lactiferous ducts
   d. Nipple

5. Gonadotropic hormones are released by the pituitary gland under the regulation of the:
   a. adrenal glands
   b. hypothalamus
   c. thalamus
   d. thyroid

6. Which pituitary hormone stimulates the ovary to produce estrogen during the menstrual cycle?

   a. FSH
   b. GnRH
   c. LH
   d. human chorionic gonadotropin (HCG)

7. During the menstrual cycle, ovulation generally occurs at which of the following times:
   a. 7 days after the last day of menstruation
   b. 14 days after the last day of the menstrual cycle
   c. 7 days before the end of menstruation
   d. 14 days before the end of the menstrual cycle

8. Variations in the length of the menstrual cycle are due to variations in the number of days in which of the following phases?
   a. Follicular phase
   b. Luteal phase
   c. Ischemic phase
   d. Secretory phase

9. A client asks, "How much blood do I lose during menstruation?" Which of the following would be the nurse's *best* response?
   a. "Normal blood loss can be a little or a lot."
   b. "Normal blood loss is about ¼ cup."   *excessive*
   c. "Normal blood loss is about 1 cup."
   d. "Normal blood loss is about ⅛ cup."   *scant*

---

For additional questions, see
*Lippincott's Self-Study Series* Software
Available at your bookstore

# ANSWER KEY

1. **Correct response: b**
   Days 6 through 14 are the proliferative phase of the menstrual (endometrial) cycle. During this phase, estrogen level is high, and the uterine lining is thick.
   a. Estrogen is not a phase of the menstrual cycle. It is a a hormone produced by the ovaries.
   c. During the luteal phase, days 15 through 22 of the ovarian cycle, the corpus luteum develops.
   d. The secretory phase, days 14 through 26 of the endometrial cycle, follows release of the ovum. During this phase, the progesterone level is high.
   *Comprehension/Safe Care/Assessment*

2. **Correct response: c**
   The uterus contains the perimetrium, myometrium, and the endometrium.
   a. The decidua is the mucous lining of the uterus during pregnancy.
   b. The ovaries are female sex glands located on each side of the uterus.
   d. The vagina, also called the birth canal, is a tubular organ lying between the rectum and the urethra.
   *Comprehension/Physiologic/Assessment*

3. **Correct response: b**
   The perineum is the tissue lying between the vaginal orifice and the anus.
   a. The mons pubis is fatty tissue over the symphysis pubis.
   c. The hymen is the membranous tissue circling the vaginal introitus.
   d. The vestibule is the area between the labia minora.
   *Knowledge/Physiologic/Assessment*

4. **Correct response: a**
   Acini cells in the breast are responsible for milk production.
   b. The areola is the pigmented area around the nipple.
   c. Lactiferous ducts in the breast transport milk to the nipple.
   d. The nipple is the raised pigmented area of the breast that lies in the center of the areola.
   *Knowledge/Physiologic/NA*

5. **Correct response: b**
   The hypothalamus controls pituitary release of gonadotropic hormones.
   a. The adrenal gland, located on the surface of the kidney, produces adrenocorticoid hormones.
   c. The thalamus lies deep within the brain just above the brain stem. It receives and deciphers sensory information.
   d. The thyroid lies in the front of the neck and controls body metabolism.
   *Knowledge/Physiologic/NA*

6. **Correct response: a**
   FSH is a pituitary hormone that stimulates the ovary to develop ovarian follicles that secrete estrogen.
   b. GnRH is a hormone released by the hypothalamus.
   c. LH is a hormone released by the anterior pituitary, which acts with FSH to cause ovulation and enhance development of the corpus luteum.
   d. HCG is a hormone secreted by the placenta, which stimulates the ovaries to produce estrogen and progesterone to maintain a healthy pregnancy.
   *Knowledge/Safe Care/Assessment*

7. **Correct Response: d**
   During the menstrual cycle, ovulation generally occurs on day 14 of a 28-day cycle. This is 14 days before the end of the menstrual cycle.
   **a, b, and c.** These responses are incorrect.
   *Knowledge/Physiologic/Assessment*

8. **Correct response: a**
   Variation in the follicular phase affects the length of the menstrual cycle.
   **b, c, and d.** These responses are incorrect.
   *Comprehension/Safe Care/Assessment*

**9.** *Correct response: c*

Normal blood loss during menstruation is about 50 mL or about ¼ cup.

**a.** This response is too vague and provides no useful information for the client.

**b.** One cup, or 240 mL, is excessive blood loss.

**d.** One-eighth cup, or 30 mL, is scant blood loss.

*Application/Physiologic/Implementation*

# Fetal Growth and

# Development

**3**

I. **Conception**
   A. Fertilization
   B. Hormones of fertilization and pregnancy
   C. Multiple pregnancy
II. **Stages of growth and development**
   A. Essential concepts
   B. Pre-embryonic stage
   C. Embryonic stage
   D. Fetal stage
   E. Amniotic fluid
   F. Placenta
III. **Genetic principles**
   A. Chromosome structure
   B. Chromosomal inheritance
   C. Chromosomal disorders (rearrangement)

IV. **Genetic counseling**
   A. Goals
   B. Screening for genetic traits and disease
   C. Indications for prenatal genetic screening
V. **Implications for nursing management**
   A. Assessment
   B. Nursing diagnoses
   C. Planning and Implementation
   D. Evaluation
   **Bibliography**
   **Study questions**

## I. Conception
### A. Fertilization

 1. Fertilization refers to impregnation as a result of the union of an ovum (egg) and a spermatozoan (sperm).

2. Following ejaculation into the vagina, sperm live approximately 48 to 72 hours but are believed to be healthy and highly fertile for only about 24 hours. Ova are considered fertile for about 24 hours after ovulation.

 3. **Thus, for fertilization to occur, coitus must be accomplished no more than 24 hours before or after ovulation.**

4. Fertilization occurs in the ampulla (outer one-third) of the fallopian tube following ovulation.

**B. Hormones of fertilization and pregnancy**

1. Estrogen: Increased levels during ovulation have three functions:
   a. Increase the fallopian tube's ability to contract and move the ovum down the tube
   b. Cause thinning of cervical mucus, facilitating sperm penetration
   c. Stimulate growth of uterine muscle (myometrium) and glandular epithelium (endometrium) and induce the synthesis of receptors for progesterone

2. Progesterone
   a. Acts on estrogen-primed endometrium to convert it to actively secreting tissue
   b. Promotes thickening and increased viscosity of cervical mucus (the mucus plug) to protect the fetus against invading bacteria
   c. Decreases motility of oviducts and uterus
   d. Stimulates growth of glandular breast tissue

3. Hormones from corpus luteum: The corpus luteum supplies most of the estrogen and progesterone in the first 2 gestational months. The persistence of the corpus luteum in supplying these hormones is essential for sustaining the uterine endometrium and preventing menstruation.

4. Human chorionic gonadotropin (HCG)
   a. Secreted by the blastocyst (the early product of conception) and the placenta, HCG is partly responsible for maintaining the corpus luteum.
   b. Detecting HCG in urine or plasma is the objective of most pregnancy tests.

5. Estriol
   a. A major estrogen of pregnancy
   b. Synthesized in the presence of a fetal adrenal enzyme
   c. Complex changes in hormone levels, basis for diagnostic tests of fetal maturity and well being

**C. Multiple pregnancy**

1. Approximately 2% of births in the United States are multiple. Most involve twins; triplets occur in 1 of 7,600 pregnancies. Multiple births higher than triplets are rare, but the incidence is rising due to the increasing use of gonadotropins to treat women with ovulatory failure.

2. **Dizygotic (fraternal) multiple pregnancy involves two or more ova fertilized by separate sperm.** Fetuses have separate placentas, amnions, and chorions (although the placenta may

fuse to resemble a single one) and may be the same or different sexes.

 **3. Monozygotic (identical) multiple pregnancy develops from a single fertilized ovum.** Fetuses share a common placenta and chorion but have separate amnions; they are the same sex and have the same genotype (Fig. 3-1).

## II. Stages of growth and development

### A. Essential concepts

1. Factors influencing embryonic and fetal development include:
   a. Environment (eg, poverty; malnutrition; maternal alcohol or drug use, including nicotine; anticoagulants and aspirin; anticonvulsants; antibiotics)
   b. Anatomic problems

      ▸ Maternal (eg, ectopic pregnancy, uterine abnormality, retroversion of uterus, incompetent cervical os)
      ▸ Fetal (eg, chromosomal defect, poor implantation)

   c. Maternal complications (eg, infection, Rh incompatibility, cyanotic heart disease, renal diseases, hypertension, urinary tract infection)
   d. Fetal complications (eg, premature rupture of membranes, preterm labor, postmaturity)
   e. Physiologic problems (eg, folate deficiency, endocrine deficiency, defective sperm)
2. Fetal development occurs in three stages: pre-embryonic, embryonic, and fetal. (Table 3-1 shows fetal development by gestational month.)

### B. Pre-embryonic stage

1. Encompassing the first 14 days after conception, this stage is characterized by rapid growth and differentiation and establishment of embryonic membranes and germ layers.

 **2. The blastocyst implants approximately 7 to 9 days after fertilization.**
3. Endometrium becomes the decidua following conception and implantation.
4. Two membranes form to protect and support the embryo:
   a. Chorion, the outside embryonic membrane
   b. Amnion, the innermost membrane
5. All tissues and organs develop from the three primary germ layers of the embryo:
   a. Ectoderm: central nervous system; peripheral nervous system; sensory epithelium of ear, nose, eye, sinus, mouth, and anal canal; skin (epidermis), hair, nails, sebaceous

*(text continued on page 36)*

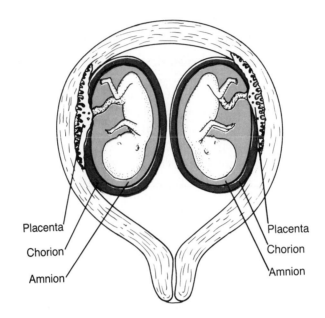

Placenta
Chorion
Amnion

Placenta
Chorion
Amnion

**A. Fraternal twins**

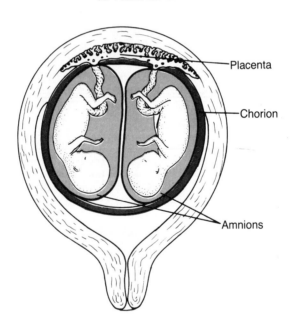

Placenta

Chorion

Amnions

**B. Identical twins**

**FIGURE 3–1.**
Among the distinctions of multiple pregnancies are the distributions of placenta, chorion, and amnions. Dizygotic (fraternal) twins (**A**) have their own placenta, chorion and amnion. Monozygotic (identical) twins (**B**) also share a placenta and a chorion but have their own amnion. (Courtesy of Reeder SJ, Martin LI, Koniak D. *Maternity Nursing,* 17th ed. Philadelphia: J.B. Lippincott, 1992).

TABLE 3-1.
Milestones in Fetal Development

| LUNAR MONTH (28 DAYS) | SIZE (LENGTH AND WEIGHT) | DEVELOPMENTAL MILESTONES |
|---|---|---|
| **1** | 0.75–1 cm<br>400 mg | Trophoblasts embed in decidua.<br>Chorionic villi form.<br>Beginnings of nervous system, genitourinary system, skin, bones, lungs, eyes, ears, and nose form. Buds of arms and legs form. |
| **2** | 2.5 cm<br>20 g | Fetus is bent.<br>Developing brain is responsible for large head formation.<br>Sex differentiation begins.<br>Bone centers begin to ossify. |
| **3** | 6–9 cm<br>45 g | Fetal fingers and toes are distinct.<br>The placenta and fetal circulation are complete. |
| **4** | 12 cm<br>110 g | Sex is differentiated.<br>Rudimentary kidneys produce urine.<br>Fetal heartbeat is present.<br>Nasal septum and palate close. |
| **5** | 19 cm<br>300 g | Lanugo covers fetal body.<br>Fetal movements can be felt by mother.<br>Heart sounds can be auscultated. |
| **6** | 23 cm<br>630 g | Fetal skin wrinkles, and vernix caseosa appears.<br>Eyebrows and fingernails develop. |

(continued)

TABLE 3-1. (continued)

| LUNAR MONTH (28 DAYS) | SIZE (LENGTH AND WEIGHT) | DEVELOPMENTAL MILESTONES |
|---|---|---|
| **7** | 27 cm 1,100 g | Fetal skin is red. Pupillary membrane disappears from eyes. Normal fetus has excellent chance of survival. |
| **8** | 28–30 cm 1,800 g | Fetus is viable. Eyelids are open. Fingerprints are set. Vigorous fetal movement occurs. |
| **9** | 32 cm 2,500 g | Fetal face and body have a loose wrinkled appearance resulting from deposit of subcutaneous fat. Lanugo disappears. Amniotic fluid decreases. |
| **10** | 36 cm 3,000–3,600 g | Skin is smooth. Eyes are slate colored. Skull bones are ossified and nearly joined at sutures. |

*Note: All measures are approximate and vary according to standard values used by practitioner and healthcare agency. (Art courtesy of Reeder SJ, Martin LL, Koniak D. Maternity Nursing, 17th ed. Philadelphia: JB Lippincott, 1992)*

        glands, sweat glands, hair follicles; and mammary glands, pituitary gland, enamel of teeth and oral glands

    b.    Mesoderm: bone, cartilage, skeleton; connective tissue, smooth and striated muscles; cardiovascular and lymphatic systems; blood and lymph cells; kidneys and reproductive organs; subcutaneous tissues of the skin; serous membrane lining of the pericardial, pleural, and peritoneal cavities; and spleen

c. Endoderm: respiratory tract epithelium, epithelial lining of gastrointestinal tract (pharynx, tongue, tonsils, thyroid, parathyroid, thymus), epithelial lining of urinary bladder and urethra, liver, and pancreas

**C. Embryonic stage**

1. This stage begins during the third week after conception and continues until embryo reaches a crown-to-rump length of 3 cm (1.2 in), about the eighth week.
2. This is the period of differentiation of tissues into organs and development of main external features.

**D. Fetal stage**

1. The period from 8 to 10 weeks after conception marks the end of the embryonic period and beginning of the fetal period.
2. At this time, every structure is present that will be found in the full-term newborn.
3. The remainder of the gestational period is devoted to refinement of structures and organization and perfection of function.

**E. Amniotic fluid**

1. Contained by the amnion that protects the embryo and fetus, this fluid controls temperature, supports symmetrical growth, prevents adherence to amnion, and allows the embryo or fetus to move within the amniotic cavity.

**2. Amniotic fluid volume normally ranges from 500 to 1,000 mL.**

**F. Placenta**

1. The placenta begins to function by the fourth week of gestation; by the 14th week, it is a complete, independently functioning organ.
2. It transmits nutrients and oxygen to the fetus and removes waste and carbon dioxide by diffusion.
3. The endocrine organ of pregnancy, the placenta, produces:
   a. HCG in maternal blood by day 8 of gestation; positive pregnancy test
   b. Human placental lactogen or human chorionic somatomammotropin; increases after 20 weeks of gestation
   c. Estrogen, which is responsible for enhancing growth of all organs; ensures nourishment and proliferation
   d. Progesterone, which maintains uterine lining for implantation, relaxes uterine smooth muscle, develops acini cells in preparation for lactation

# III. Genetic principles

## A. Chromosome structure

 1. **Normal embryonic cell tissue contains 46 chromosomes (23 pairs): 44 homologous (22 pairs) and 2 sex (1 pair) chromosomes.**

2. Each chromosome contains 22 autosomes and 1 sex chromosome (Y) from the male and 22 autosomes and 1 sex chromosome (X) from the female.

 3. **Human life begins as a single cell, zygote, that reproduces itself (as does each new cell).**

4. Fetal cells and organs develop from chromosomes; the sex of the embryo is determined from the one pair (two sex chromosomes, one from each parent); female is XX, and male is XY.

5. The sex of the fetus is determined at the time of fertilization by the combination of the sex chromosomes of the sperm (X or Y) and the ovum (Fig. 3-2).

6. Usually by the 12th week of gestation, external genitalia are developed enough to be easily distinguishable.

7. In a female fetus, the fetal ovary has many primordial (primitive) follicles and produces small but increasing amounts of estrogen.

8. The gonads of the genetically male fetus (fetus with Y chromosome) play a critical role in forming the genital tract. As the gonads evolve in the testicular pattern—presumably under the influence of maternal HCG and luteinizing hormone (LH) and fetal adrenal hormones—the testes produce androgenic hormones that promote growth and differentiation of male genitalia.

## B. Chromosomal inheritance

1. *Basic patterns of single-gene inheritance include:*

   a. *Autosomal dominant:* the clinical expression of a mutant gene in a heterozygous (one allele—an alternate form of

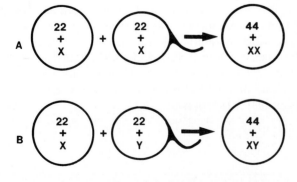

FIGURE 3–2.
Fetal sex is determined genetically at fertilization. (**A**) Ovum fertilized by sperm bearing X chromosome will form a female zygote. (**B**) Ovum fertilized by sperm bearing Y chromosome will form a male zygote.

a gene—at a given chromosome locus) individual. Disorders include achondroplastic dwarfism

b. *Autosomal recessive:* the clinical expression of a mutant gene when both alleles at a given chromosome locus are mutant (homozygous). Disorders include cystic fibrosis.

c. *X-linked dominant:* rare disorders appearing in every generation of a family. Females, having two X chromosomes, will be symptomatic if heterozygous for an X-linked dominant trait. Males, having only one X chromosome and a Y chromosome, will always be affected if they inherit an X-linked mutant gene.

d. *X-linked recessive:* females will be asymptomatic for a trait if heterozygous for an X-linked recessive trait. Females will manifest symptoms if homozygous for an X-linked recessive disorder. (Note: the terms dominant and recessive in X-linked traits refer only to females.)

 2. **Multifactorial inheritance involves traits and disorders resulting from the interaction of many genetic factors** (polygenetic inheritance) or the interaction of genetic and environmental factors. Examples of multifactorial disorders include congenital heart defects, clubfoot, neural tube defects, pyloric stenosis, cleft lip and cleft palate, and congenital hip dysplasia.

C. **Chromosomal disorders (rearrangement)**

1. Causes may be hereditary or nonhereditary; contributing factors include internal and external events, such as exposure to radiation, certain drugs, viruses, toxins and chemicals, and advanced maternal age at conception.

2. Types include:

a. Numeric abnormalities in sex chromosomes and autosomes (eg, Klinefelter's and Turner's syndromes and trisomy 13, 18, or 21)

b. Structural disorders, such as deletions (eg, cri du chat syndrome) and translocations, which are aberrations that result when part of a chromosome is transferred to a different chromosome

**IV. Genetic counseling**

A. **Goals**

1. Enables individuals or couples to make informed reproductive decisions

2. Provides psychological support for decision-making

3. Provides clients with information about the defect in question

4. Communicates to clients the risk of transmitting the defect in question to future children

**B.** **Screening for genetic traits and disease**

1. The goal of screening is to prevent tragic genetic diseases and offer various reproductive options to at-risk couples.

2. Accurate screening hinges on the education and advocacy of physicians and nurses caring for people of reproductive age and on accurate identification of the client's ethnic origin.

3. Specific tests include:

   a. *Newborn blood analysis:* obtained by heelstick within 3 to 5 days of birth to detect phenylketonuria, maple syrup urine disease, galactosemia, homocystinuria, tyrosinemia, and hypothyroidism

   b. *Maternal serum alpha-fetoprotein (MSAFP) screen:* selectively done when an open neural tube defect is suspected (MSAFP is not diagnostic; there is, however, a 5% to 10% risk of the defect when MSAFP is elevated at 16 to 18 weeks' gestation.)

   c. *Triple screening:* analysis of three indicators from maternal serum—alpha fetoprotein, estriol, and human chorionic gonadotropin—which yields more reliable results than MSAFP

   d. *Heterozygote screening:* directed at detecting clinically normal carriers of a disease-causing mutant gene, particularly in people of ethnic groups with high frequency of the mutant gene under investigation, for example, Tay-Sachs disease in Jews of Eastern European (Ashkenazi) descent, sickle-cell disease in people of African descent, and beta-thalassemia (Cooley's anemia) in people of Mediterranean descent (eg, Italian, Turkish, Sicilian, Sardinian, Greek, Cypriotic)

**C.** **Indications for prenatal genetic screening**

1. Risk factors for chromosomal disorders, such as:

   a. Advanced maternal age

   b. Known carrier parent

   c. Previous birth of child with chromosomal disorder or with multiple anomalies with no chromosomal studies done

   d. History of spontaneous abortion

2. Known risk for metabolic disorders

3. Known risk for sex-linked genetic disorder

4. Willingness to interrupt pregnancy if abnormal fetus is detected

**V.** **Implications for nursing management (Note: See Chapter 8, Antepartal Care, for information on assessing fetal growth and development.)**

**A.** Assessment: Obtain a relevant preliminary genetic history, being alert to information indicating the need for referral to genetic counseling.

**B.** Nursing diagnoses
1. Decisional Conflict
2. Anticipatory Grieving
3. Knowledge Deficit
4. Body Image Disturbance

**C.** Planning and implementation
1. Identify families who need genetic counseling.
2. Provide sufficient and correct information about the genetic problem in question.
3. Serve as a liaison between the genetic counselor and the family.
4. Assist families in coping with the information received; guide them in managing the crisis in their lives.

**D.** Evaluation
1. Couples of childbearing age from any setting are appropriately screened for genetic problems and given appropriate referrals.
2. Families faced with difficult decisions with respect to genetic outcomes state that they receive adequate information.
3. Families of childbearing age have access to anticipatory guidance and information.
4. The psychological adaptation of family members to grief and loss related to genetic problems is documented in the nursing process.

## *Bibliography*

Bobak, I. M., & Jensen, M. D. (1993). *Maternity and gynecologic care: The nurse and the family* (5th ed.). St. Louis: C.V. Mosby.

May, K. A., & Mahlmeister, L. R. (1994). *Maternal and neonatal nursing: Family centered care* (3rd ed.). Philadelphia: J.B. Lippincott.

Olds, S. B, London, M. L., & Ladewig P. W. (1992). *Maternal-newborn nursing: A family centered approach* (4th ed.). Menlo Park, CA: Addison-Wesley.

Reeder, S. J., Martin L. L., & Koniak, D. (1992). *Maternity nursing: Family, newborn, and women's health care* (17th ed.). Philadelphia: J.B. Lippincott.

## STUDY QUESTIONS

1. The thickened endometrium in which the fertilized embryo implants is called the:
   a. endoderm
   b. decidua
   c. amnion
   d. chorion

2. The fetal nervous system is formed by the germ layer known as the:
   a. ectoderm
   b. mesoderm
   c. endoderm
   d. entoderm

3. The corpus luteum acts as the placenta for the implanted ovum until:
   a. the end of the first gestational month
   b. the end of the fifth gestational month
   c. the end of the fourth gestational month
   d. the end of the second gestational month

4. An expectant mother in the prenatal clinic stated. "I'm sure I'm going to have a boy because my husband says he knows it's a boy." Which of the following would be the nurse's best response?
   a. "You could be right."
   b. "The female determines the sex of the newborn."
   c. "There are more girls born than boys."
   d. "The male determines the sex of the newborn."

5. If a client expelled a 19-cm fetus, which of the following would be the approximate gestational age of the fetus?
   a. 3 months
   b. 5 months
   c. 2 months
   d. 4 months

6. Which of the following substances is measured when a neural tube defect is suspected?
   a. Estrogen
   b. Progesterone
   c. Alpha-fetoprotein
   d. LH

7. The placenta transports nutrients and oxygen to the fetus by:
   a. capacitation
   b. diffusion
   c. fertilization
   d. ustulation

8. An expectant mother asks the nurse in the prenatal clinic, "When can I expect to feel my baby move?" The nurse's best response would be:
   a. at about 2 months
   b. at about 3 months
   c. at about 4 months
   d. at about 5 months

9. An expectant mother in the prenatal clinic informs the nurse that she smokes and asks if she could continue to do so. Which of the following would be the *best* response?
   a. "How much do you smoke each day?"
   b. "You should decrease the number of cigarettes you smoke."
   c. "Outside factors, such as smoking and alcohol use, may adversely affect your baby's development. Women who smoke have smaller babies than nonsmokers."
   d. "That is something you should ask the physician."

10. An expectant mother in the prenatal clinic confides that she has frequent headaches and has always taken aspirin. Which of the following would be the *best* response?
    a. "Did you take aspirin in the first 4 weeks of your pregnancy?"
    b. "The physician may recommend another medication for your headaches."
    c. "Could you tell me more about these headaches and when you get them?"
    d. "We do not recommend using any medication during pregnancy."

# ANSWER KEY

**1.** *Correct response: b*
The fertilized ovum implants in the decidua.
**a.** This is a germ layer.
**c. and d.** These structures form the placenta.
*Knowledge/Physiologic/Assessment*

**2.** *Correct response: a*
The ectoderm forms the fetal nervous system.
**b.** The mesoderm forms muscles, bone, cartilage, teeth dentin, ligaments, tendons, kidneys, heart, and other structures.
**c.** The endoderm forms the epithelium of the digestive tract and respiratory tract.
**d.** This is another name for the endoderm.
*Knowledge/Physiologic/Assessment*

**3.** *Correct response: d*
By the end of the second gestational month, the placenta is functional.
**a, b, and c.** these responses are incorrect.
*Knowledge/Physiologic/Assessment*

**4.** *Correct response: d*
The male determines the sex of the fetus.
**a.** This is a nonprofessional response, and it offers no instruction.
**b.** This is an incorrect statement.
**c.** Although this statement is correct, it is not the most appropriate response to the client's statement.
*Comprehension/Physiologic/
Implementation*

**5.** *Correct response: b*
The average fetal length at 5 months' gestation is 19 cm.
**a.** 6 to 9 cm long = 3 months.
**c.** 2.5 cm long = 2 months.
**d.** 12 to 17 cm long = 4 months.
*Comprehension/Physiologic/Assessment*

**6.** *Correct response: c*
MSAFP screening is selectively done when an open neural tube defect is suspected.
**a and b.** These hormones work together to maintain pregnancy and promote fetal well-being.
**d.** LH, which stimulates follicular growth, is an incorrect response.
*Analysis/Physiologic/Analysis (Dx)*

**7.** *Correct response: b*
Most nutrients and oxygen move across the placenta by diffusion.
**a.** Capacitation refers to changes in the ovum that facilitate penetration by the sperm.
**c.** Fertilization refers to impregnation by the union of an ovum and a sperm.
**d.** Ustulation refers to drying of a moist drug by heat.
*Knowledge/Physiologic/NA*

**8.** *Correct response: d*
At about 5 gestational months, fetal movements are usually felt by the mother. At this time, the average fetus is about 19 cm long and weighs about 300 g.
**a, b, and c.** On average, these are all too early for the mother to sense defined movement.
*Comprehension/Physiologic/Assessment*

**9.** *Correct response: c*
Smoking during pregnancy has been proven to increase the risk of a developmental problem, especially small-for-gestational age newborn.
**a and b.** These responses may be helpful, but neither is the best response in this situation.
**d.** The nurse can intervene independently of the physician in this situation.
*Application/Physiologic/Implementation*

**10.** *Correct response: c*

With this response, the nurse keeps in mind the possible developmental complications related to medication use while seeking additional information about the characteristics and frequency of the headaches.

**a.** This is an inappropriate response because it would alarm the client.

**b.** This statement may be true: however, it does not yield information about the headaches, which may impact on the quality of care given to the mother and newborn.

**d.** This response is too restrictive.

*Application/Physiologic/Implementation*

# Infertility

## I.  Overview

### A.  Fertility

1.  The reproductive potential of men and women depends on multiple factors, including age, sex, and overall health status.

2.  See Chapters 2 and 3 for discussions of fertility and conception.

### B.  Infertility

1.  Infertility is the inability to conceive after at least 1 year of regular sexual intercourse without contraception.

2.  Primary infertility means having no previous history of either partner conceiving or impregnating.

3.  Secondary infertility is the inability to conceive after a previous successful pregnancy.

4.  Although infertility implies that some potential for conception exists, sterility denotes a total and irreversible inability to become pregnant or to impregnate.

### C.  Incidence of infertility

1.  In the last 30 years in the United States, infertility has decreased from 11% to 8%.

2. Under optimal conditions, about 20% of couples who try to conceive will do so within 1 month.

 3. **Infertility results from a problem for the woman 40% of the time; a problem for the man 40% of the time; a problem for both 10% of the time; and an unidentified cause 10% of the time.**

**D.** **Etiology**

1. Causes of female infertility include:

   a. Vaginal problems include vaginal infections, anatomic abnormalities, sexual dysfunction that prevents penetration by the penis, a highly acidic vaginal environment, which markedly decreases sperm survival.

   b. Cervical problems can involve a disruption in any of the physiologic changes that normally occur during the preovulatory and ovulatory period that make the cervical environment conducive to sperm survival (eg, opening of the cervical os, increased alkalinity, increased secretions, ferning); mechanical problems include cervical incompetence associated with women whose mothers were treated with diethylstilbestrol (DES) during pregnancy.

   c. Uterine problems may be functional (eg, an unfavorable environment for the movement of sperm up the uterus into the fallopian tubes or for implantation after fertilization) or structural (eg, uterine myomas or leiomyomas).

   d. Tubal causes are becoming more prominent with the increased incidence of pelvic inflammatory disease (PID), which leads to scarring that obstructs the fallopian tubes; the increased use of intrauterine devices (IUDs) contributes to the rise in PID, because 40% of infections associated with IUD use are asymptomatic and remain untreated. Endometriosis also can contribute to tubal obstruction.

   e. Ovarian problems include anovulation, oligo-ovulation, and polycystic ovary syndrome; secretory malfunctions also contribute (eg, inadequate progesterone secretion or an inadequate luteal phase will interfere with the ability for a fertilized ovum to be maintained).

2. Causes of male infertility include:

   a. Congenital factors (eg, maternal history of DES ingestion during pregnancy, absence of the vasa deferentia or the testes)

   b. Ejaculation problems (eg, retrograde ejaculation associated with diabetes, nerve damage, medications, or surgical trauma)

   c. Sperm abnormalities (eg, inadequate sperm production

or maturation, inadequate motility, blockage of sperm along the male reproductive tract, or inability to deposit sperm in the vagina)

 d. Testicular abnormalities due to illness (eg, orchitis associated with mumps after puberty), cryptorchidism, trauma, or irradiation

 e. Coital difficulties related to obesity or spinal nerve damage

 f. Drugs (eg, methotrexate, amebicides, sex hormones, and nitrofurantion) that interfere with spermatogenesis

 g. Other factors that interfere with sperm or semen production, including infections (eg, sexually transmitted diseases), stress and inadequate nutrition, excessive alcohol intake, and nicotine

**3.** Interactive problems resulting from causes specific to the couple, such as:

 a. Insufficient frequency of sexual intercourse

 b. Poor timing of intercourse

 c. Development of antibodies against a partner's sperm

 d. Use of potentially spermicidal lubricants, such as petroleum jelly and some water-soluble lubricants

## II. Diagnostic evaluation of infertility

 **A.** Initial assessment

  **1.** **Evaluation of infertility begins with physical examination of both partners and basic laboratory tests, including complete blood count, thyroid function tests, and urinalysis.**

  2. If these results are negative, an infertility work-up consisting of more intensive tests begins.

 **B.** Diagnostic studies

  1. Semen analysis

   a. The test is performed after 48 to 72 hours of abstinence from orgasm to avoid false low readings.

   b. Repeated serial analysis is done 74 days apart.

   c. Sperm count, volume of ejaculate, infection, seminal viscosity, and presence or absence of agglutination of sperm are considered.

  2. Postcoital test

   a. Couple is instructed to have sexual intercourse at the presumed time of ovulation after a 48-hour period of abstinence.

   b. Immediately after intercourse, a sample of cervical mucus is examined microscopically to detect characteristics that enhance sperm survival and to assess adequacy of estrogen production.

**3.** Basal temperature recordings
   a. For several cycles, the woman takes and records oral temperatures daily when awakening.
   b. A biphasic pattern with persistent temperature elevation for 12 to 14 days before menstruation indicates that ovulation has occurred.
**4.** Serum progesterone test or endometrial biopsy
   a. A blood sample is drawn during the presumed luteal phase of the menstrual cycle.
   b. An adequate progesterone level suggests that ovulation has probably occurred. (The normal serum progesterone level is 10 ng/mL or higher, with a lower level of 3 to 4 ng/mL at an earlier stage of the luteal phase.)
   c. Endometrial biopsy provides direct histologic information about the endometrial tissue.
   d. If adequate secretory tissue is identified, secretion of progesterone and luteinizing hormone is normal, indicating that ovulation has occurred.
**5.** Hysterosalpingography
   a. Radiopaque dye is injected through the cervix into the uterus. Fluoroscopy shows whether the fallopian tubes fill with dye.
   b. A radiograph is taken 24 hours later to determine if the dye has dispersed in the pelvic cavity, an indication of fallopian tube patency.
   c. The study must be done after menstruation has ceased to prevent the possibility of old menstrual blood being pushed into the tubes and causing infection.
   d. The study also must be done before ovulation to prevent pushing a fertilized ovum out through the fimbrial end of the tubes.
**6.** Other tests
   a. Immunoassays of semen and male or female serum to determine if antibody formation against the partner's sperm is a factor in infertility
   b. Sperm penetration assay, an in vitro test to determine the ability of the sperm to penetrate the zona pellucida of the ova from superovulated hamsters

**III.** **Medical management of infertility**
   **A.** **Fertilization techniques**
      **1.** In vitro fertilization
         a. This technique is used when damaged or obstructed fallopian tubes impair transport of a fertilized egg to the uterus.
         b. The first recorded success was in 1978 in England.

    c.    Following a course of medication (eg, Pergonal) to stimulate ovulation, the ovary is punctured during laparoscopy, and mature follicles are removed by suction.

    d.    Each egg is incubated for several hours in a sugar, salt, and protein mixture designed to simulate maternal fluids found in the fallopian tubes.

    e.    Semen is added, and the eggs and fluid are again incubated; if the egg is fertilized, it is incubated further until cell division begins, at which time the fertilized egg is deposited in the woman's uterus using a thin plastic catheter.

**2.** Surrogate embryo transfer (SET)

    a.    This is used when the woman cannot produce normal mature follicles, and the male partner is fertile.

    b.    The first child resulting from SET was born in 1984.

    c.    Using hormonal therapy, the menstrual cycles of the donor and the recipient woman are synchronized.

    d.    Sperm of the fertile partner is artificially inseminated in the fertile donor following her normal ovulation.

    e.    Several days after fertilization occurs, the fertilized egg is washed from the donor's uterus and deposited in the recipient's uterus; if successful, implantation occurs soon afterward.

**3.** Gamete intrafallopian tube transfer

    a.    An ovum is surgically retrieved from the ovary and implanted into the fallopian tube.

    b.    Sperm are then implanted into the fallopian tube.

    c.    Fertilization may then occur naturally.

**4.** Zygote intrafallopian tube transfer

    a.    The ovum is fertilized externally.

    b.    The fertilized zygote is then returned to the fallopian tube by an instrument such as a laparoscope.

**4.** In vivo fertilization or embryo transplantation

    a.    This is indicated when the recipient woman cannot conceive naturally but can carry a fetus to maturity.

    b.    An embryo conceived in one woman is transplanted into the uterus of another.

    c.    Genetically, the fetus is the result of the union of the man's sperm with the ovum of the donor woman.

**5.** Surrogate mothering

    a.    This is used when a woman is not only unable to conceive, but also is unable to carry a fetus to viability.

    b.    Semen from the partner is artificially inseminated into the host (surrogate mother).

    c.    After birth, the newborn is given to the infertile couple.

           d.    Legislation is pending in many states to regulate this practice.

**B.** **Other treatments**

    1.   Medical interventions include:

        a.   Altering acidic cervical mucus by having the woman douche with an alkaline solution 30 minutes before intercourse

        b.   Removing environmental hazards associated with oligospermia (eg, tight underclothes, hot tubs or saunas, certain drugs, chemicals, and toxins)

    2.   Surgical interventions may include:

        a.   Correction of anatomic defects and removal of obstructions in the female reproductive tract (eg, removal of uterine fibroid tumors, cerclage of an incompetent cervix, microsurgery to open blocked fallopian tubes)

        b.   Ligation of varicocele in the man

    3.   Pharmocologic interventions can include:

        a.   Antibiotic therapy to treat infections

        b.   Testosterone to treat oligospermia

        c.   Estrogen therapy to increase the abundance of cervical mucus and enhance ferning and spinnbarkeit

        d.   Ovulation-induction medications to treat anovulation

**C.** **Sexual therapy**

    1.   This therapy for infertility involves treatment of sexual problems that may interfere with conception (eg, vaginismus or dyspareunia without an identifiable organic, physical, or mechanical cause and psychogenic impotence).

    2.   One approach to sex counseling involves gathering assessment data on a couple's sexual difficulties, then clarifying each member's perceptions of the other and of sexual activities in general.

    3.   The therapist facilitates communication between the two partners and their acceptance of each other's feelings and attitudes.

    4.   The couple may be taught specific exercises and different coital positions to assist in increasing control during sexual activity or enjoyment in the pleasure of sex.

**IV.** **Implications for nursing management**

  **A.**   **Assessment**

    1.   Evaluate the couple's sexual and reproductive history to rule out sexual dysfunction as a cause of infertility.

    2.   Assess the couple's knowledge of sexuality, sexual techniques, and infertility.

    3.   Perform a complete physical examination, and arrange for appropriate diagnostic and laboratory tests for both partners.

    4.   Assess the following:

        a.   The couple's general lifestyle, including use of medicines,

drugs, and other substances; nutrition; exercise and rest patterns
  b.  The couple's usual strategies for coping with stress and anxiety
  c.  The couple's psychosocial responses associated with infertility—stage of emotional healing, cultural influences, belief systems, and effect on self-image

**B.  Nursing diagnoses**
  1.  Ineffective Family and Individual Coping
  2.  Knowledge Deficit
  3.  Body Image Disturbance
  4.  Sexual Dysfunction
  5.  Spiritual Distress

**C.  Planning and implementation**
  1.  Keep in mind that diagnosis and treatment of infertility typically occurs over several years and represents a significant financial and emotional commitment.
  2.  Assist the couple to regain a sense of control by:
      a.  Using stress-reduction techniques
      b.  Pointing out successes and achievements in other areas of their lives

*m*  **3.  Provide advocacy and support for decision-making:**
      a.  **Listen nonjudgmentally and facilitate decision-making.**
      b.  **Allot time to talk about ideas, concerns, issues of conflict.**
      c.  **Provide access to other sources and networks for information and support.**
      d.  **Offer referral to appropriate agencies.**
  4.  Provide anticipatory guidance:
      a.  Explain the complex battery of diagnostic tests.
      b.  Discuss protocols of fertility evaluation.
      c.  Point out responses to such procedures and the impact on sexual functioning and the couple's relationship.

*m*  **5.  Provide accurate information, and dispel myths associated with infertility that foster guilt, self-doubt, and feelings of inadequacy.**
  6.  Help the couple resolve their feelings about infertility.

**D.  Evaluation**
  1.  The infertile couple demonstrates positive adjustment to the demands of the diagnostic and treatment regimens.
  2.  The infertile partners verbalize their individual and collective feelings related to infertility, diagnosis, and treatment.
  3.  The infertile couple exhibits evidence of healthy coping mechanisms when dealing with infertility.

## Bibliography

Bobak, I. M., & Jensen, M. D. (1993). *Maternity and gynecologic care: The nurse and the family* (5th ed.). St. Louis: C.V. Mosby.

May, K. A., & Mahlmeister, L. R. (1994). *Maternal and neonatal nursing: Family Centered care* (3rd ed.). Philadelphia: J.B. Lippincott.

Olds, S. B., London, M. L., & Ladwig, P. W. (1992). *Maternal-newborn nursing: A family centered approach* (4th ed.). Menlo Park; CA: Addison-Wesley.

Reeder, S. J., Martin, L. L., & Koniak, D. (1992). *Maternity nursing: Family, newborn, and women's health care* (17th ed.). Philadelphia: J.B. Lippincott.

# STUDY QUESTIONS

1. A couple has been trying to conceive for 2 years. Their records reveal no physiologic problem that would prevent conception. General information provided to the couple to increase the likelihood of conception by optimal timing of intercourse would not include which of the following:
   a. Ovulation usually occurs 14 days before the onset of the menstrual cycle.
   b. An ovulated egg has a lifespan of 12 to 24 hours.
   c. The male's abstinence from ejaculation for 73 to 96 hours increases the likelihood of conception.
   d. Ejaculated sperm have a lifespan of 24 to 48 hours.

2. A couple has one child. They have been trying, without success, for several years to have another child. Their situation would be referred to as:
   a. primary infertility
   b. secondary infertility
   c. irreversible infertility
   d. viable infertility

3. When assessing the adequacy of sperm for conception to occur, which of the following is the most useful criterion?
   a. Sperm count
   b. Sperm motility
   c. Sperm maturity
   d. Semen volume

4. A client who is seeking help in becoming pregnant reveals that her mother took DES while her mother was pregnant with the client. Which of the following would be the most accurate analysis of this information?
   a. It is of concern because maternal use of DES is linked to PID in female offspring.
   b. It is of concern because maternal use of DES is linked to cervical incompetence in female offspring.
   c. It is of no concern because use of DES is *not* linked to any problems in offspring.
   d. It is of no concern because maternal use of DES is linked to reproductive problems in male offspring.

5. The client's medical history includes a ruptured appendix and resulting peritonitis. Why might these data be pertinent to the client's infertility problems?
   a. Scarring and adhesions may have created anatomic deformities or tubal blocking.
   b. The infection may have caused sterility.
   c. The appendix is important to tubal functioning.
   d. Surgical removal of the appendix is likely to sever the fallopian tubes.

6. A couple wants to conceive but has been unsuccessful during the last 3 years. They have undergone many diagnostic procedures. When discussing the situation with the nurse, one partner states, "All the couples we know in our age group are having their second or third child, yet we are so inadequate that we can't even produce one. With our luck, we'd probably have a defective baby anyway." The most pertinent nursing diagnosis for this couple would be:
   a. Fear related to the unknown
   b. Altered Comfort related to numerous procedures
   c. Ineffective Family Coping related to infertility
   d. Self Esteem Disturbance related to infertility

7. An infertile couple has never used contraception and usually has intercourse three to four times a week. Both independently express a high degree of sexual satisfaction. They practice some sexual experimentation with position, time, and location, and they use petroleum jelly for additional lubrication. The man's sperm count is lower than nor-

mal, but other assessment data appear to be well within normal limits. Based on these data, the nurse's recommendation for potentially increasing the likelihood of conception would include which of the following?

a. Advise the couple to reduce frequency of intercourse to once a week. WILL NOT

b. Advise them to be more consistent in how they have intercourse.

c. Instruct them to stop using the additional lubrication.

d. Clarify the validity of their sexual satisfaction.

**8.** Introduction of radiopaque material into the uterus and fallopian tubes to assess tubal patency is known as:

a. uterotubal insufflation

b. laparoscopy

c. culdoscopy

d. hysterosalpingography

**9.** The results of various diagnostic procedures indicate serious problems for a man with a low sperm count and a woman with fibroid tumors blocking the fallopian tubes. Both partners begin to laugh when one says, "Oh, we were so worried nothing could be done to help us begin a family. We'll just take care of these two things, and then we'll have a baby." The couple's reaction to the seriousness of their fertility problem most likely indicates which of the following?

a. Denial of the seriousness of the problem

b. Concealed anger with each another

c. Joyful relief toward the seriousness of the problem

d. Coping with a positive attitude

**10.** Desperately desiring children, a couple has spent 10 years undergoing numerous procedures. Each partner has had corrective surgery. Both have accepted marital therapy to help them cope with anger and disappointment. Today they reveal that they have decided to adopt a child. While discussing their decision with the nurse, they are smiling and holding hands. The man says. "I'm glad I'll never have to see this place [the fertility clinic] again." Based on this information. The nurse would most accurately evaluate their behavior as an indication of:

a. denial of their chance to have their own child

b. anger at the nurse for wasting their time

c. apathy concerning their state of infertility

d. acceptance of infertility

---

For additional questions, see
*Lippincott's Self-Study Series* Software
Available at your bookstore

# ANSWER KEY

1. **Correct response: c**
   Abstinence normally has no effect on conception.
   **a, b, and d.** These statements are all accurate.
   *Comprehension/Safe Care/ Implementation*

2. **Correct response: b**
   Because the couple successfully conceived previously, their situation would be accurately described as secondary infertility.
   **a.** Primary infertility would apply if the couple had never conceived a child.
   **c.** No information in this scenario suggests irreversible infertility (sterility).
   **d.** This is an incorrect term in reference to infertility.
   *Comprehension/Physiologic/Analysis (Dx)*

3. **Correct response: b**
   Although all of the factors listed are important, sperm motility is the most significant criterion when assessing male infertility.
   **a, c, and d.** Sperm count, sperm maturity, and semen volume are all significant, but they are not as significant as sperm motility.
   *Knowledge/Physiologic/Analysis (Dx)*

4. **Correct response: b.**
   Maternal use of DES has been linked to cervical abnormalities in female offspring.
   **a, c, and d.** These responses are incorrect.
   *Comprehension/Safe Care/Assessment*

5. **Correct response: a**
   Scarring and adhesions are possible, because of this client's history.
   **b and d.** These problems are highly unlikely.
   **c.** This is an untrue statement.
   *Application/Physiologic/Analysis (Dx)*

6. **Correct response: d**
   The data presented most likely support self-esteem issues as the couple's primary problem.
   **a, b, and c.** These diagnoses also may apply to this couple as secondary issues.
   *Application/Psychosocial/Diagnosis*

7. **Correct response: c**
   Petroleum jelly and some water-soluable lubricants have been shown to be spermicidal.
   **a.** Reducing the frequency of intercourse will not increase the probability of conception.
   **b and d.** The information presented does not indicate that these are factors in this couple's inability to conceive.
   *Analysis/Safe Care/Implementation*

8. **Correct response: d**
   Only hysterosalpingography involves a radiopaque material.
   **a, b, and c.** None of these procedures use radiopaque material.
   *Comprehension/Safe Care/Assessment*

9. **Correct response: a**
   Denial is a typical initial reaction to "bad news" that allows time for adjusting to a threatening situation.
   **b.** Although the couple may be angry with each other, no data support this analysis.
   **c and d.** This situation involves neither joy nor positive feelings.
   *Analysis/Psychosocial/Analysis (Dx)*

10. **Correct response: d**
    The couple is demonstrating acceptance of their situation by taking steps to obtain children despite their infertility.
    **a and b.** This couple's history of 10 years of therapeutic assistance indicates that they have moved through anger and denial.
    **c.** They have not demonstrated apathy and resignation but have made every effort to achieve conception.
    *Analysis/Psychosocial/Evaluation*

# Family Planning and Contraception

## I. Overview

### A. Family planning

 1. Family planning is the conscious process by which a couple decides on the number and spacing of children and the timing of births.

2. Specific objectives of family planning include:

 a. **Avoiding unwanted pregnancies through contraception**

b. Regulating intervals between pregnancies

c. Deciding the number of children in the family

d. Controlling the time at which births occur

e. Preventing pregnancy for women with serious illness in whom pregnancy would pose a health risk

f. Providing the option of avoiding pregnancy to women who are carriers of genetic disease

3. The overall goal of nursing intervention in family planning is to improve general maternal, neonatal, and family health.

4.   Preconception planning—an ideal that is not always real-
           ized—offers couples an opportunity to enhance the proba-
           bility of having a healthy newborn. It involves examining
           the health history and physical health of both partners and
           providing appropriate instruction relative to physical, psy-
           chological, and financial preparation for pregnancy and
           childbirth.

**B.** Nursing care
   1.   Assisting the couple to select and use an effective contraceptive
        method is an important part of the nurse's role.
   2.   Understanding one's own philosophy, beliefs, and standards is
        important to avoid presenting biased information.
   3.   Informing the individual or couple about the complete range
        of contraceptive possibilities is a key factor in helping the client
        make an informed and satisfactory contraceptive choice.
   4.   Understanding and teaching about current available contracep-
        tive methods and their use, effectiveness, advantages, disadvan-
        tages, and side effects are vital nursing roles in reproductive
        healthcare.

      5.   **Providing an understanding, comfortable, factual, non-
           judgmental attitude when discussing contraception and
           sexuality is a significant element of effective nursing care.**
   6.   Compiling a thorough health history and assessment data is es-
        sential to planning appropriate contraception teaching.

**C.** Contraception
   1.   Contraception is the voluntary prevention of pregnancy. The
        decision to practice contraception has individual and social im-
        plications.
   2.   When choosing an appropriate contraceptive method, the
        client must consider many factors, including:
        a.   Religious orientation
        b.   Social and cultural values
        c.   Medial contraindications
        d.   Psychological contraindications
        e.   Individual sexual expression
        f.   Cost
        g.   Availability of bathroom facilities and privacy
        h.   Partner's support and willingness to cooperate
        i.   Personal lifestyle

      3.   **The best contraceptive method is the one that is the most
           comfortable and natural for the partners and the one that
           they will use correctly and consistently.**

**4.** Contraceptive effectiveness is defined in terms of maximal effectiveness and typical effectiveness:

    a. Maximal effectiveness: a method's effectiveness under ideal conditions (ie, when completely understood and used as recommended)

    b. Typical effectiveness: a method's effectiveness under actual use, in which some people use the method correctly and others use it carelessly or incorrectly

## II. Contraceptive methods

### A. Natural or fertility awareness methods

    **1.** Calendar method

        a. The calendar (rhythm) method relies on abstinence from intercourse during fertile periods.

        b. Fertile periods are calculated by recording 12 consecutive menstrual cycles, then subtracting 18 days from the end of the shortest cycle and subtracting 11 days from the end of the longest cycle to determine the fertile period

        c. Advantages: It is inexpensive and convenient, has no side effects, encourages communication, is ethically and morally noncontroversial, and is appropriate for sex education programs.

        d. Disadvantages: In general, it requires long periods of abstinence and self-control, correct calculations, and regular menstrual periods to be effective; confusing irregular uterine bleeding with a menstrual period may lead to incorrect calculations. Effectiveness is unreliable and depends on many variables.

    **2.** Basal body temperature (BBT) method

        a. Contraception by the BBT method uses the single sign of a rise in BBT to predict ovulation (signaling the fertile period) and to begin abstinence. In general, abstinence begins with the first days of menses and continues until the third day of temperature elevation.

        b. BBT is measured by taking and recording the temperature orally or rectally each morning before arising. BBT drops before ovulation and rises 0.4 to 0.8°F with ovulation (in response to progesterone production from the corpus luteum).

        c. Advantages: It is inexpensive, has no side effects, encourages communication, is ethically and morally noncontroversial, and is appropriate for sex education programs.

        d. Disadvantages: It is not as effective as other methods; temperature elevation may result from conditions other than ovulation; requires regular and accurate record keeping; and calls for partner to have intercourse only in the postovulatory period (usually about 10 days of the month).

3. Cervical mucus method
   a. This method uses the appearance, characteristics, and amount of cervical mucus to identify ovulation. Because of the activity of estrogen and progesterone in the ovulatory period, cervical mucus is clear and slippery (like an egg white) and more abundant. In the preovulatory and postovulatory periods, cervical mucus is yellowish, less abundant, and thick and sticky, thereby inhibiting sperm motility.
   b. Advantages: It is inexpensive, has no side effects, and is not controversial.
   c. Disadvantages: It is not as effective as other methods.

4. Symptothermal method
   a. The couple uses a combination of the above techniques to determine the fertile period.
   b. Advantages: It is inexpensive, provides couple with more information, encourages communication, and has no side effects.
   c. Disadvantages: It is more complex and difficult to learn and requires regular and daily effort.

5. Mittelschmerz
   a. Between menstrual cycles, some women experience pain when the ovary releases an egg. Rarely, the pain may be accompanied by scant vaginal spotting. Some couples may use this symptom to signal the beginning of the fertile period.
   b. Advantages: It is convenient and inexpensive.
   c. Disadvantages: It requires reliable and identifiable pain and differentiation between like symptoms; it is not as reliable as other methods.

**B. Coitus interruptus**
   1. This method requires withdrawal of the penis from the vagina before ejaculation.
   2. It is highly ineffective because sperm exist in pre-ejaculatory fluid.
   3. Advantages: It is inexpensive and medically safe.
   4. Disadvantages: It is unreliable, interrupts sexual excitation or plateau, and diminishes satisfaction.

**C. Spermicides**
   1. Vaginal jelly, cream, suppository, or foam preparations interfere with sperm viability and prevent sperm from entering the cervix.
   2. They are nearly 80% effective.

3. Advantages: They are available without prescription, useful when other methods are inappropriate or contraindicated, and have few or no side effects.
4. Disadvantages: They have a lower effectiveness than other methods; may irritate tissues (most products contain alum); and are esthetically unpleasant. The couple must remember to apply within 30 minutes before intercourse, reapply before each subsequent coitus, and avoid douching for 8 hours after intercourse.

**D.  Barrier methods**
   1. Female condom (vaginal pouch)
      a. This is a long polyurethane sheath that inserts manually into the vagina with a flexible internal ring forming the cervical barrier and a wide outer ring extending to cover the perineum; it is lubricated with spermicide (nonoxynol-9).
      b. It is about 85% effective.
      c. Advantages: It protects against sexually transmitted diseases (STDs) and conception, allows woman to control protection, is inexpensive for single use, and is disposable.
      d. Disadvantages: It is esthetically unappealing, requires dexterity, is expensive for frequent use, may cause sensitivity to sheath material, and decreases spontaneity.
   2. Male condom
      a. This is a rubber sheath that fits over the erect penis that prevents sperm from entering vagina.
      b. It is about 88% effective.
      c. Advantages: It helps prevent conception and transmission of STDs, is available without prescription, and has no side effects.
      d. Disadvantages: It may decrease spontaneity, may decrease sensation, and should be used with vaginal jelly if condom or vagina is dry.
   3. Cervical cap
      a. This is a small rubber or plastic dome that fits snugly over the cervix.
      b. It is about 82% effective.
      c. Advantages: Plastic cap can remain in place for 3 to 4 weeks; rubber cap can remain in place 24 to 36 hours. (Valvular cap, which is not approved for use in the United States, may stay in place for up to 1 year.)
      d. Disadvantages: It may dislodge, must be filled with spermicide, must be fitted individually by a health care provider, and may not be used if woman has anatomic abnormalities or allergy to plastic, rubber, or spermicide.

      e.    Side effects: Trauma to cervix or vagina, pelvic infection, cervicitis, or abnormal Pap test results are possible.

   4.   Diaphragm

      a.    This is a flexible ring covered with a dome-shaped rubber cap that inserts into the vagina and covers the cervix. It is used with spermicide in dome and around the rim and is applied no more than 2 hours before intercourse and left in place for 6 hours after coitus with additional spermicide applied for repeated intercourse.

      b.    Estimates of effectiveness vary between 82% and 94%.

      c.    Advantages: It is reusable and inexpensive with use over several years.

      d.    Disadvantages: It requires dexterity to insert and must be fitted individually and refitted after childbirth or after a weight loss of 15 lb or more.

      e.    Side effects: Toxic shock syndrome, cystitis, cramps or rectal pressure, allergy to spermicide or rubber are possible.

**E.   Intrauterine device (IUD)**

   1.   This is a flexible device inserted into the uterine cavity where it causes a localized sterile inflammatory reaction.

   2.   Estimates of effectiveness vary between 93% (typical effectiveness) and 97% (maximal effectiveness).

   3.   Advantages: It is inexpensive for long-term use and requires no attention other than checking that it is in place (by feeling for attached string in vaginal canal).

   4.   Disadvantages: There are possibly serious side effects. It is available only through a health care provider and cannot be used if woman has active or chronic pelvic infection, postpartum infection, endometrial hyperplasia or carcinoma, or uterine abnormalities.

   5.   Side effects: Dysmenorrhea, increased menstrual flow, spotting between periods, uterine infection or perforation, and ectopic pregnancy are possible. Danger signs to report to health care provider include late or missed menstrual period, severe abdominal pain, fever and chills, foul vaginal discharge, and spotting, bleeding, or heavy menstrual periods.

**F.   Pharmacologic methods**

   1.   Oral contraceptives

      a.    Combined estrogen and progesterone preparation in tablet form inhibits the release of FSH, LH, and an ovum. They are taken daily and are available in numerous hormone combinations (and as progesterone-only preparation). Biphasic and triphasic contraceptives closely mirror hormonal fluctuations of the menstrual cycle.

b. They are about 97% effective.

c. Advantages: They are among the most reliable contraceptive methods and are convenient to use.

d. Disadvantages: They should not be used by women who smoke; have a history of thrombophlebitis, circulatory disease, varicosities, diabetes, estrogen-dependent carcinomas, liver disease; or are older than 35 years. Reassessment and reevaluation are essential every 6 months.

e. Side effects: Breakthrough bleeding, nausea, vomiting, susceptibility to vaginal infections, thrombus formation, edema, weight gain, irritability or missed periods are possible. Danger signs indicating complications include abdominal pain, chest pain or shortness of breath, headaches, blurred or loss of vision, leg pain in calf or thigh.

2. Subdermal implants

a. These consists of six soft implanted Silastic rods filled with synthetic progesterone that leaks into bloodstream. They inhibit ovulation, making cervical mucus hostile to sperm, and inhibiting implantation in the endometrium and are known as Norplant.

b. Estimates of effectiveness vary from 0.04% failure to 99% effective within 24 hours (dropping to 96% effective after 5 years).

c. Advantages: They are long acting (effective for up to 5 years), reversible, inexpensive over life of drug, and require little attention other than health care visits for problems or scheduled health maintenance.

d. Disadvantages: They require surgical insertion through a half-inch incision on the inside surface of the nondominant arm. They may be difficult to remove and should not be used by a woman who has active thrombophlebitis, unexplained bleeding, active liver disease or tumor, or known or suspected breast cancer.

e. Side effects: Tenderness and bruising at the insertion site, irregular bleeding, headaches, acne, weight change, breast tenderness are possible. Signs of reportable complications include infection, bleeding, or pain at insertion site; subdermal rod breaking through skin; heavy vaginal bleeding; severe abdominal pain; and sudden menstrual irregularity after a regular cycle has been established.

3. Subcutaneous injections

a. Medroxyprogesterone (DMPA or Depo-Provera) is injected every 3 months; it works like subdermal implant.

b. Effectiveness is similar to subdermal implant.

      c.    Advantages: It is highly effective and requires little attention except for returning to health care provider for injection every 3 months.

      d.    Disadvantages are similar to those for subdermal implants; risk for breast cancer and osteoporosis may be increased.

      e.    Side effects are similar to those for subdermal implants but primarily spotting, headache, and weight gain.

**G.**  **Sterilization**

    1.  Vasectomy

      a.    Surgical ligation of the vas deferens terminates sperm passage through the vas completely after residual sperm clear the male reproductive tract.

      b.    It is almost 100% effective (nurses should point out finality of procedure).

      c.    Advantages: It is highly effective and usually permanent.

      d.    Disadvantages: It requires surgery and may be irreversible, although reversal success rates vary (anatomic success, 40%–90%; clinical success 18%–60%).

    2.  Tubal ligation

      a.    The fallopian tubes are surgically ligated or cauterized.

      b.    It is almost 100% effective (nurses should stress finality of procedure).

      c.    Advantages: It is highly effective and usually permanent.

      d.    Disadvantages: It requires invasive procedure and may be irreversible, although tubal reconstruction has a 50% to 70% successful reversal rate.

**III.**  **Implications for nursing management**

    **A.**  **Assessment**

      1.  Determine the type of contraception the woman or couple desires.

      2.  Obtain a thorough medical, surgical, menstrual, and obstetric history to identify any contraindications to the desired method.

      3.  Perform a precontraception physical examination to include breast and pelvic examination, vital signs measurements, and other aspects as appropriate.

      4.  Arrange for and evaluate results of appropriate precontraception laboratory tests (eg, Pap smear, serologic test for syphilis, culture for gonorrhea, urinalysis, and complete blood count).

    **B.**  **Nursing diagnoses**

      1.  Altered Health Maintenance

      2.  Knowledge Deficit

      3.  Self Care Deficit

      4.  Decisional Conflict

      5.  Spiritual Distress

**C.** **Planning and implementation**

1. Evaluate the woman's or couple's knowledge of available contraceptive methods; provide information to correct misconceptions.
2. Assist the woman or couple in choosing an appropriate method.
3. Teach the woman or couple about the chosen method, including, as appropriate:
    a. Insertion and removal (eg, diaphragm)
    b. Application and removal (eg, condom)
    c. Dosage schedule for oral contraceptives
    d. Techniques for natural methods
4. Discuss possible side effects and steps to take if they occur.

**D.** **Evaluation**

1. **The woman or couple verbalizes satisfaction with the selected contraceptive method.**
2. The woman or couple demonstrates accurate understanding of how to use the selected method.
3. The woman or couple verbalizes any danger signs associated with the method selected.

## Bibliography

Bobak, I. M., & Jensen, M. D. (1993). *Maternity and gynecologic care: The nurse and the family* (5th ed.). St. Louis: C.V. Mosby.

May, K. A., & Mahlmeister, L. R. (1994). *Maternal and neonatal nursing: Family-centered care* (3rd ed.). Philadelphia: J.B. Lippincott.

McElmurry, B. J., & Parker, R. S. (Ed.). (1993). *Annual review of women's health.* New York: National League for Nursing.

Olds, S. B., Lonoon, M. L., & Ladewig, P. W. (1992). *Maternal-newborn nursing: A family-centered approach* (4th ed.). Menlo Park, CA: Addison-Wesley.

Pillitteri, A. (1995). *Maternal and child health nursing: Care of the childbearing family* (2nd ed.). Philadelphia: J.B. Lippincott.

Reeder, S. J., Martin, L. L., & Koniak, D. (1992). *Maternity nursing: Family, newborn, and women's health care* (17th ed.). Philadelphia: J.B. Lippincott.

## STUDY QUESTIONS

1. Which of the following methods of contraception would be most appropriate for a breast-feeding mother for the first 6 weeks after birth?
   a. Birth control pills
   b. Estrogen injections
   c. An IUD
   d. Condom and spermicidal foam

2. Of the following methods of contraception, which is likely to be the least effective for most couples?
   a. Intrauterine device
   b. Coitus interruptus
   c. Subdermal implant
   d. Condom and foam

3. The diaphragm must be refitted after childbirth or after a weight loss of:
   a. 10 lb
   b. 15 lb
   c. 8 lb
   d. 5 lb

4. The IUD prevents pregnancy by:
   a. altering the environment in the fallopian tubes
   b. altering the environment in the endometrium
   c. altering the speed at which the ovum travels
   d. an unknown mechanism of action

5. Which of the following statements best describes natural family planning?
   a. In natural family planning, the couple may choose any birth control method but must practice it consistently.
   b. Natural family planning requires rare periods of abstinence to be effective.
   c. Natural family planning relies on recognizing the body's signs and symptoms of fertility.
   d. Natural family planning is indicated when the safest, most effective method is desired.

6. Among the following, the most effective means of contraception is generally considered to be:
   a. spermicidal jelly or cream
   b. the intrauterine device
   c. the rhythm method
   d. a postcoital vaginal douche

7. When advising a 35-year-old woman who has given birth to her third child and who smokes one pack of cigarettes per day, the nurse would most likely recommend which of the following contraceptive methods?
   a. Coitus interruptus
   b. Birth control pills
   c. A tubal ligation
   d. Intrauterine device

8. A postpartum teenaged mother confides, "I will never have sex again." Which of the following would be the nurse's best response to her statement?
   a. "That's a good decision, and I approve of it."
   b. "Usually people who have had sexual experience want to continue."
   c. "Learning about contraception may be a good plan so that you can be in control."
   d. "If your school has a sex education course, you should enroll in it."

9. A woman using a diaphragm for contraception should be advised to leave it in place for how long after intercourse?
   a. 1 hour
   b. 12 hours
   c. 28 hours
   d. 6 hours

10. Uterine infection, uterine perforation, and ectopic pregnancy are complications associated with which of the following contraceptive methods?
    a. IUD
    b. Contraceptive pills
    c. Subdermal implants
    d. Cervical cap

# ANSWER KEY

1. **Correct response: d**
   The condom with spermcidal foam is safest for the breast-feeding mother and newborn during the first 6 weeks after birth.
   **a and b.** Estrogen and progesterone cross over into breast milk.
   **c.** A woman can resume intercourse earlier than 6 weeks after birth, but the IUD or diaphragm cannot be fitted until 6 weeks after the birth.
   *Application/Safe Care/Planning*

2. **Correct response: b**
   Coitus interruptus is withdrawal of the penis from the vagina before ejaculation occurs. It is highly ineffective because there are sperm in pre-ejaculatory fluid.
   **a.** The IUD has a typical effectiveness of 93%.
   **c.** Subdermal implants are highly effective over a long period.
   **d.** Cervical caps are effective if used correctly and consistently.
   *Comprehension/Health Promotion/ Planning*

3. **Correct response: b**
   The diaphragm must be refitted after childbirth or if there is a weight loss of 15 lb.
   **a, c, and d,** These are incorrect responses.
   *Comprehension/Health Promotion/ Planning*

4. **Correct response: b**
   The IUD is a foreign body and initiates a sterile inflammatory response, which prevents implantation of a fertilized ovum.
   **a and c.** These mechanisms are not known to occur.
   **d.** This is an incorrect response.
   *Analysis/Physiologic/Analysis (Dx)*

5. **Correct response: c**
   Natural family planning relies on the self-discipline of the couple in recognizing the body's signs and symptoms of fertility.
   **a, b, and d.** These are incorrect responses.
   *Analysis/Physiologic/Assessment*

6. **Correct response: b**
   Of those methods listed, the IUD is the most effective.
   **a.** Spermicides are effective but not as effective as the IUD.
   **c.** Natural rhythm methods can be effective for women with regular menstrual cycles, but they are not as effective as the IUD.
   **d.** Douching is the most ineffective of the methods listed.
   *Analysis/Health Promotion/Planning*

7. **Correct response: d**
   Of the methods listed, the IUD is the most effective except for sterilization.
   **a.** Coitus interruptus is not very effective for any woman.
   **b.** Oral contraceptives are not given to older women who smoke because of the risk of embolism.
   **c.** The nurse would not recommend sterilization because of its permanency.
   *Analysis/Safe Care/Planning*

8. **Correct response: c**
   Research has demonstrated that adolescents respond better to contraceptive teaching when they believe that they are in control.
   **a.** This is a judgmental response, so it is not appropriate.
   **b.** This is true, as proven by research.
   **d.** This is an inappropriate response.
   *Analysis/Health Promotion/ Implementation*

9. **Correct response: d**
   The diaphragm should remain in place at least 6 hours after intercourse and no more than 12 hours to avoid the possibility of toxic shock syndrome.

**a, b, and c.** These responses are incorrect.

*Analysis/Safe Care/Implementation*

**10.** *Correct response: a*
Uterine infection, uterine perforation, and ectopic pregnancy are complications associated with the IUD.

**b, c, and d.** These responses are incorrect.

*Comprehension/Health Promotion/Analysis (Dx)*

# Biopsychosocial Aspects
# of Pregnancy

6

## I. Biophysical aspects of pregnancy

  **A.** Overview

     **1.** All maternal body systems are altered by pregnancy.

     **2.** Such changes are normal, inevitable, and temporary.

  **B.** Signs and symptoms of pregnancy

     **1.** Presumptive (subjective) changes include:

        a. Amenorrhea

        b. Nausea and vomiting

        c. Urinary frequency

        d. Breast tenderness and changes

        e. Excessive fatigue

     **2.** Probable (objective) changes include:

        a. Changes in pelvic organs:

> ▶ Goodell's sign: softening of the cervix
> ▶ Hegar's sign: softening of isthmus of uterus
> ▶ Ladin's sign: soft spot anteriorly in middle of the uterus
> ▶ McDonald's sign: flexibility of the uterus against the cervix
> ▶ Piskacek's sign: enlargement and softening of the uterus

    b. Enlargement of abdomen

    c. Uterine souffle (soft, blowing sound at rate of maternal pulse)

    d. Changes in skin pigmentation

    e. Quickening (maternal perception of fetal movement)

 **3. Positive (diagnostic) changes include:**

    **a. Fetal heart beat: audible at 10 to 12 weeks' gestation by Doppler ultrasound and 16 to 20 weeks' gestation with a fetoscope (normal fetal heart rate, 120–160 beats/min)**

    **b. Fetal movements palpable by examiner**

    **c. Ultrasonography confirming presence of fetus**

    **d. Fetal electrocardiography recording fetal heart pattern**

**C. Reproductive system changes**

    **1.** Uterus

        a. Uterine growth:

> ▶ Length: from 2½ in to 12½ in
> ▶ Width: from 1½ in to 9½ in
> ▶ Depth: from 1 in to 8½ in
> ▶ Weight: from 2½ oz to 2½ lb
> ▶ Volume: from 1 to 2 mL to 5,000 mL

        b. Enlargement results from increasing size of myometrial cells.

        c. Hyperplasia of uterine muscle fibers occurs in the first 6 weeks of pregnancy. Hypertrophy of uterine muscle fibers and dilation of uterine blood vessels causes uterine enlargement after the first trimester.

        d. Increased fibrous tissue adds strength and elasticity to the uterine muscle wall.

        e. Uterine circulatory requirements increase; accordingly, so do the size and number of blood vessels and lymphatics.

        f. Braxton Hicks contractions (painless contractions) occur intermittently throughout pregnancy and can be felt by the woman by the fourth month.

         **g. Normal uterine growth—measured in terms of fundal height—is evaluated in relation to other anatomic structures. After 20 weeks' gestation, fundal height in**

centimeters approximates the weeks of pregnancy up to 36 weeks.

2. Cervix
   a. Glandular tissue is stimulated by estrogen.
   b. Endocervical glands secrete thick mucus that forms a mucous plug.

    c. **The mucus plug seals the endocervical canal and prevents contamination of uterus by bacteria and other substances.**
   d. The mucus plug is expelled when cervix begins to dilate.
   e. Goodell's sign results from increased cervical vascularization.

3. Ovaries
   a. They do not produce ova during pregnancy.
   b. Corpus luteum, which develops from ruptured follicle, produces hormones (estrogen and progesterone) for 10 to 12 weeks of pregnancy, then regresses by midpregnancy.

4. Vagina and external genitalia
   a. Increased vascularization causes tissue to thicken and soften.
   b. Increased vascularization of vagina causes a blue-purple coloration (Chadwick's sign).
   c. Vaginal discharge tends to be thick, white, and acidic (pH, 3.5–6.0).

5. Breasts
   a. Breast size increases, and breasts become more nodular due to glandular hyperplasia and hypertrophy.
   b. The nipple and areola darken; superficial veins become more prominent.
   c. Striae may develop in late pregnancy.

    d. **Colostrum may leak or be expressed from the breast during the last 3 months of pregnancy.**

D. **Respiratory system changes**
   1. The diaphragm elevates, and substernal angle increases due to an enlarging uterus.
   2. Displacement of diaphragm causes shortness of breath.
   3. Nasal stuffiness and epistaxis are common due to edema and vascular congestion induced by increased estrogen.
   4. Respiratory rate increases by about two breaths per minute, and vital capacity increases slightly; breathing more deeply increases the efficiency of gas exchange. However, functional residual capacity and residual volume are decreased due to elevation of the diaphragm.

**E.** **Cardiovascular system changes**
1. Heart is displaced upward, to the left, and forward.
2. Blood volume increases 45% during pregnancy; red blood cell volume increases 20% to 30%; hematocrit decreases 7%, causing physiologic anemia of pregnancy; fibrin level may increase as much as 40%; and leukocytes increase.
3. Pulse rate increases 10 to 15 beats/min.
4. Blood pressure decreases slightly, then returns to near normal during the third trimester.
5. As uterus enlarges, pressure on blood vessels increases, possibly caused increased pressure and edema in the leg veins.

6. **Supine hypotensive syndrome during the second trimester may be caused by pressure of enlarged uterus on the vena cava when the woman lies supine.**

**F.** **Gastrointestinal system changes**
1. Nausea and vomiting frequently occur during the first trimester.
2. Gum tissue may become soft and bleed when traumatized.
3. Secretion of saliva may increase.
4. Gastric acidity decreases. Heartburn and flatulence may result due to the reduction in gastric acidity, growing uterus, and smooth muscle relaxation.
5. Bloating and constipation may occur due to delayed gastric emptying time and decreased intestinal motility.

**G.** **Urinary system changes**
1. Urine output increases; urine-specific gravity decreases.
2. Dilation of the kidneys and urethra may occur, especially on the right side, due to the pressure of the enlarged uterus.
3. Urinary stasis and urinary tract infections may occur due to dilated uterus.
4. The woman is at increased risk for glycosuria.
5. Urinary frequency occurs in the first and third trimesters due to pressure from the enlarged uterus.

**H.** **Integumentary system changes**
1. Pigmentation changes occur in the areola, nipple, vulva, perianal area, and linea alba.
2. Facial chloasma (mask of pregnancy) and vascular spider nevi may develop.
3. Striae (stretch marks) commonly appear on the abdomen, breasts, and thighs.
4. Activity of sebaceous and sweat glands may increase.

**I.** **Skeletal system changes**
1. Sacroiliac, sacrococcygeal, and pubic joints relax during pregnancy.

    **2.** Symphysis pubis may separate slightly.

    **3.** Lumbodorsal spinal curve is increased during the third trimester, commonly producing low back pain.

**J. Metabolic changes**

    **1.** Metabolism accelerates during pregnancy.

    **2. Average weight gain is 24 to 30 lb,** which is comprised of:

      a. Fetus: 7½ lb

      b. Placenta and membrane: 1½ lb

      c. Amniotic fluid: 2 lb

      d. Uterus: 2½ lb

      e. Breasts: 3 lb

      f. Increased blood volume: 2 to 4 lb

      g. Extravascular fluid and fat: 4 to 9 lb

    **3. Increased water retention is a basic chemical alteration of pregnancy.**

      a. Contributory factors include increased level of steroid sex hormones affecting sodium and fluid retention, lowered serum protein, and increased intracapillary pressure and permeability (normal increase is about 7 L of fluid).

      b. Fetus, placenta, and amniotic fluid account for 3.5 L of fluid.

      c. Increased blood volume, interstitial fluid, and hypertrophied maternal organs account for 3.5 L of fluid.

**K. Endocrine system changes**

    **1.** Thyroid: increase in vascularity and hyperplasia; rise in thyroxin ($T_4$); and 25% increase in basal metabolic rate

    **2.** Parathyroid: concentration of hormone secreted and size of gland increases.

    **3.** Pituitary

      a. Slight hypertrophy during pregnancy

      b. Anterior pituitary: prolactin responsible for beginning lactation after delivery

      c. Posterior pituitary: releases oxytocin (to produce uterine contractions) and vasopressin (to promote vasoconstriction and antidiuretic effect)

    **4.** Adrenals

      a. The adrenals undergo little structural change.

      b. Cortisol levels regulate metabolism of carbohydrates and proteins.

    **5.** Pancreas: increased insulin production

    **6. Placenta**

      a. **Endocrine gland of pregnancy**

      b. **Secretes human chorionic gonadotropin (HCG), estrogen, and progesterone**

7.  Hormones of pregnancy
    a.  HCG: produced by the chorion; stimulates corpus luteum to produce estrogen and progesterone
    b.  Human placental lactogen: increases circulating free fatty acids for maternal metabolism
    c.  Estrogen: stimulates development of uterine environment suitable for fetus (increases uterus' size and weight and augments blood supply)
    d.  Progesterone: maintains endometrium and decreases contractility of the uterus
    e.  Relaxin: decreases uterine activity and softens the cervix

**L.  Nutrition during pregnancy**
1.  Hormonal effects on nutrition stem from:
    a.  Progesterone, which causes relaxation of the smooth muscle, including the gastrointestinal tract, and reduces motility, allowing more nutrients to be absorbed; increases maternal fat deposition; increases renal sodium excretion
    b.  Estrogen, which increases water retention
    c.  HCG, which is implicated in nausea
2.  Some metabolic adjustments during pregnancy are the basis for the increased nutritional requirements and dietary allowances. These include:
    a.  A 50% greater plasma volume by 34 weeks' gestation than at conception, creating an increased need to carry oxygen and nutrients
    b.  Increased serum lipid levels (triglycerides, cholesterol, free fatty acids, and vitamin A), probably due to increased circulating steroids, because cholesterol is a precursor for the synthesis of progesterone and estrogen in the placenta
    c.  Increased blood flow through the kidneys and increased glomerular filtration rate to facilitate the clearance of waste products from the woman and fetus
3.  The total energy cost of pregnancy is 80,000 calories; averaged over the entire pregnancy, it amounts to about 300 extra calories per day. Additional increases are recommended by the National Academy of Sciences (Table 6-1).
4.  Protein requirements increase to provide sufficient amino acids for fetal development, increased blood volume, and breast and uterine tissue growth; the recommended daily allowance is 30 g/d more than nonpregnant needs.
5.  Pregnancy increases requirements for all vitamins.
6.  **Commonly recommended nutritional supplements contain vitamins B$_6$, D, E, and C; folic acid; pantothenic acid; iron; calcium; magnesium; zinc; and copper.**

TABLE 6–1.
Average Recommended Nutritional Requirements During Pregnancy

| | PREGNANCY | NONPREGNANCY |
|---|---|---|
| **Vitamins** | | |
| A (mcg RE*) | 800 | 800 |
| B₆ (mg) | 2.2 | 1.6 (ages 19–50) |
| | | 1.5 (ages 15–18) |
| | | 1.4 (ages 11–14) |
| B₁₂ (mcg) | 2.2 | 2 |
| C (mg) | 70 | 60 (ages 15–50) |
| | | 50 (ages 11–14) |
| D (mcg) | 10 | 5 (ages 25–50) |
| | | 10 (ages 11–24) |
| E (mg TE†) | 10 | 8 |
| K (mcg) | 65 | 65 (ages 25–50) |
| | | 60 (ages 19–24) |
| | | 55 (ages 15–18) |
| | | 45 (ages 11–14) |
| Folic acid (mcg) | 400 | 180 (ages 15–50) |
| | | 150 (ages 11–14) |
| Thiamin (mg) | 1.5 | 1.1 |
| Riboflavin (mg) | 1.6 | 1.3 |
| Niacin (mg) | 17 | 15 |
| **Minerals** | | |
| Calcium (mg) | 1,200 | 800 (ages 25–50) |
| | | 1,200 (ages 11–24) |
| Iodine (mg) | 175 | 150 |
| Iron (mg) | 30 (add iron supplement to daily diet) | 15 |
| Magnesium (mg) | 320 | 280 (ages 19–50 and 11–14) |
| | | 300 (ages 15–18) |
| Phosphorus (mg) | 1,200 | 800 (ages 25–50) |
| | | 1,200 (ages 11–24) |
| Zinc (mg) | 15 | 12 |
| **Proteins** (g/d) | 76 | 46 |
| **Calories** (kcal/d) | 2,300 (ages 23–50) | 2,000 (ages 23–50) |
| | 2,400 (ages 15–22) | 2,100 (ages 15–22) |
| | 2,500 (ages 11–14) | 2,200 (ages 11–14) |

*Retinol equivalents; †Tocopherol equivalents.
Compiled from the National Academy of Sciences (1989). Recommended dietary allowances (10th ed.). Washington, DC: National Academy Press.

7.  Dietary calcium is the best way to increase calcium intake to support the growing fetus (eg, dairy products, beans, and leafy, green vegetables [collard, mustard, kale, turnip, broccoli]).

8.  Because of the mixed effects of calcium on iron and zinc absorption, daily calcium supplements exceeding 100 g are not recommended during pregnancy.

9.  Vitamin oversupplementation may lead to vitamin toxicity.

## II. Psychosocial aspects of pregnancy

### A. Overview

1.  Pregnant women tend to become more dependent, needing increased nurturing so that they can nurture their developing offspring.

2.  Pregnant women may need social service programs.

### B. Psychosocial stages of pregnancy

1.  Anticipatory stage: Women train for role of expectant parent and interact with babies and children.

2.  Honeymoon stage: They fully assume role and initially may seek help from family members.

3.  Plateau stage: The role is fully exercised; the expectant parent validates adequacy of current role.

4.  Disengagement: The termination stage precedes and includes termination of the role, in this case pregnancy, which commonly ends with labor (although it may terminate in other ways).

### C. Meaning and effect of pregnancy on couple

1.  The male partner experiences changes in perceived body space from the eighth month of gestation through the third postpartum month.

 2.  **Men also may experience physical and psychological changes during their partner's pregnancy.**

3.  The coming child represents the synthesis of three distinct entities:
    a.  Relationship of woman and partner
    b.  Relationship of woman and developing fetus
    c.  Relationship of woman and newborn

4.  The mother can never again be a single unit.

5.  Necessary tasks of pregnancy for a woman or couple include:
    a.  Belief that she is pregnant and incorporation of fetus into body image
    b.  Preparation for physical separation with birth of newborn
    c.  Resolution and identification of conflicts that accompany role transition, thus preparing for smooth functioning of family

6. Common emotional reactions to pregnancy include:
   a. First trimester: ambivalence, fear, fantasies, anxiety
   b. Second trimester: well-being, increased need to learn about fetal growth and development, narcissism, passivity, introversion (may seem egocentric and self-centered)
   c. Third trimester: feels awkward, clumsy, unattractive; becomes more introverted; reflects on own childhood

## III. Implications for nursing management (Also see Chapter 8, Antepartum Care.)

A. Assessment
   1. Begin biopsychosocial assessment at the initial prenatal visit.
   2. Perform ongoing data collection at each subsequent visit.
   3. **Make every effort to include the expectant father in the early prenatal visits.**
   4. Focus assessment on the expectant parents' adaptation to pregnancy.
   5. Evaluate for risk factors associated with poor adaptation:
      a. Prior negative childbearing or childrearing experiences
      b. Inadequate preparation for childbearing or childrearing
      c. Significant health concerns
      d. Negative response to the pregnancy
      e. Conflicts or problems in support system

B. Nursing diagnoses
   1. Anxiety
   2. Ineffective or Compromised Family or Individual Coping
   3. Altered Family Processes
   4. Fear
   5. Knowledge Deficit
   6. Altered Role Performance
   7. Self Esteem Disturbance
   8. Altered Health Maintenance
   9. Social Isolation

C. Planning and implementation
   1. Plan time to address questions and concerns of both expectant parents. This can alleviate anxiety and fear and increase understanding of roles.
   2. Provide opportunities for ongoing psychosocial and biophysical assessment.
   3. Discuss or demonstrate effective self-care measures as needed.
   4. **Offer anticipatory guidance (eg, reassure woman that nausea usually decreases; help man understand that many men**

do not feel involved in the pregnancy until the last few weeks; explain what to expect next month).

**D.** Evaluation

1. Expectant parents exhibit progress toward healthy adaptation to childbearing.
2. Expectant parents express satisfaction with increased knowledge level.
3. Expectant parents express realistic plans for the pregnancy.
4. Expectant family exhibits adequate emotional and financial support systems.

## Bibliography

Bobak, I. M., & Jensen, M. D. (1993). *Maternity and gynecologic care: The nurse and the family* (5th ed.). St. Louis: C.V. Mosby.

Gorrie, T. M., McKinney, E. S., & Murray, S. S. (1994). *Foundations of maternal newborn nursing.* Philadelphia: W.B. Saunders.

May, K. A., & Mahlmeister, L. R. (1994). *Maternal and neonatal nursing: Family-centered care* (3rd ed.). Philadelphia: J.B. Lippincott.

McElmurry, B. J., & Parker, R. S. (Ed.) (1993). *Annual review of women's health.* New York: National League for Nursing.

Olds, S. B., London, M. L., & Ladewig, P. W. (1992). *Maternal-newborn nursing: A family centered approach* (4th ed.). Menlo Park, CA: Addison-Wesley.

Reeder, S. J., Martin, L. L., & Koniak, D. (1992). *Maternity nursing: Family newborn, and women's health care* (17th ed.). Philadelphia: J.B. Lippincott.

# STUDY QUESTIONS

1. Which of the following urinary symptoms is most frequently experienced by the pregnant woman during the first trimester?
   a. Dysuria
   b. Frequency
   c. Incontinence
   d. Burning

2. Gastrointestinal discomfort, common in the second trimester, is most likely the result of:
   a. increased plasma HCG levels
   b. increased emptying time
   c. smooth muscle relaxation and uterine enlargement
   d. elevated estrogen levels

3. Chloasma is an irregular hyperpigmented area on the:
   a. breasts, areola, and nipples
   b. chest, neck, arms, and legs
   c. abdomen, breast, and thighs
   d. cheeks, forehead, and nose

4. A pregnant client states that she "waddles" when she walks. The nurse would explain that this is the result of:
   a. the large size of the newborn
   b. pressure on the pelvic muscles
   c. relaxation of the pelvic joints
   d. excessive weight gain

5. Which of the following represents optimal weight gain during pregnancy?
   a. 12 to 22 lb
   b. 15 to 25 lb
   c. 24 to 30 lb
   d. 25 to 40 lb

6. At 5 months' gestation, a woman reports that she has felt intermittent, painless, irregular, contractions of her uterus and asks the nurse about them. What would be the nurse's best response?
   a. "It is important to time these contractions, because it may be the beginning of labor."
   b. "If these contractions occur again, call your physician immediately."
   c. "The contractions help stimulate the movement of blood through the placenta."
   d. "They are called Braxton Hicks contractions. They may occur throughout pregnancy."

7. When talking with a pregnant client who is experiencing aching, swollen, leg veins, the nurse would explain that this is most probably the result of:
   a. thrombophlebitis
   b. pregnancy-induced hypertension
   c. pressure from the enlarging uterus
   d. the force of gravity on the uterus

8. During a prenatal visit, the nurse is able to feel fetal movements and auscultate the fetal heart rate with a fetoscope. These changes of pregnancy are known as:
   a. expected changes
   b. presumptive changes
   c. probable changes
   d. positive changes

9. Of the following, which is *not* a presumptive sign of pregnancy?
   a. Goodell's sign
   b. Nausea
   c. Skin pigmentation changes
   d. Positive pregnancy test

10. Which of the following common emotional reactions to pregnancy occur in the first trimester?
    a. introversion, egocentrism, narcissism
    b. feels awkward, clumsy, not pretty
    c. anxiety, passivity, extroversion
    d. ambivalence, fear, fantasies

## ANSWER KEY

80

**1.** *Correct response:* **b**

Urinary frequency is common in the first trimester, resulting from pressure and irritation of the bladder by the growing uterus.

**a, c, and d.** These are symptoms associated with urinary tract infections.

*Comprehension/Physiologic/Analysis (Dx)*

**2.** *Correct response:* c

During the second trimester, pressure from the growing uterus and smooth muscle relaxation can cause gastrointestinal discomfort.

**a.** HCG levels increase in the first trimester.

**b.** Gastric emptying time decreases in the second trimester.

**d.** Estrogen levels decrease in the second trimester.

*Comprehension/Physiologic/Analysis (Dx)*

**3.** *Correct response:* d

Chloasma is irregular hyperpigmented areas on the face.

**a, b, and c.** Chloasma is not seen on any of these areas.

*Knowledge/Safe Care/Assessment*

**4.** *Correct response:* c

Pelvic relaxation due to hormonal changes can cause a waddling gait.

**a.** The growing fetus will cause changes in posture.

**b.** A growing uterus will produce pressure on muscles and cause discomfort.

**d.** Weight gain will not affect the gait.

*Comprehension/Physiologic/Evaluation*

**5.** *Correct response:* c

Normal weight gain during pregnancy ranges from 24 to 30 pounds.

**a.** This is insufficient weight gain.

**b.** This is marginal weight gain.

**d.** This is excessive weight gain.

*Knowledge/Health Promotion/Implementation*

**6.** *Correct response:* d

Braxton Hicks contractions are a normal antepartum phenomenon that probably result from stretching of the uterine muscles.

**a.** Braxton Hicks contractions are not a sign of labor.

**b.** These contractions are normal and do not warrant notifying the physician.

**c.** These contractions have no effect on placental perfusion.

*Application/Health Promotion/Implementation*

**7.** *Correct response:* c

Pressure of the growing uterus will cause increased tendency toward blood stagnation in the lower extremities, resulting in edema and varicose vein formation.

**a.** Thrombophlebitis is an inflammation of veins due to thrombus formation.

**b.** Pregnancy-induced hypertension is not associated with these symptoms.

**d.** Gravity is only a minor factor associated with these symptoms.

*Application/Physiologic/Evaluation*

**8.** *Correct response:* d

These changes confirm pregnancy.

**a.** This is not considered a categorical change of pregnancy.

**b.** These symptoms suggest but do not confirm pregnancy.

**c.** These changes strongly suggest pregnancy but are not diagnostic.

*Comprehension/Physiologic/Assessment*

**9.** *Correct response:* b

Nausea is a presumptive sign of pregnancy.

**a, c, and d.** These are all probable signs of pregnancy.

*Knowledge/Physiologic/Assessment (Dx)*

**10.** *Correct response:* d

Common emotional reactions to the pregnancy include ambivalence, fears, and fantasies in the first trimester.

**a.** These reactions are common in the second trimester.

**b.** These reactions occur in the third trimester.

**c.** This is an incorrect response.

*Knowledge/Psychosocial/Assessment (Dx)*

# Childbirth Education

## I. Overview

### A. History of childbirth education

1. Women have always shared information about childbirth with each other. Until the late 19th century, childbirth was viewed primarily as women's work.

2. **The first formal childbirth education classes in the United States were offered by the American Red Cross in 1913, resulting from concern for public health.**

3. In 1919, the Maternity Center Association in New York began to offer childbirth education classes. However, formal classes did not become available to most expectant parents for many years.

4. Grantly Dick-Read, an English physician, published two books, *Natural Childbirth* (1933) and *Childbirth Without Fear* (1944). These works became the foundation for organized childbirth education in the United States, Canada, Great Britain, and South Africa.

5.  Specially trained nurses established the International Childbirth Education Association in 1960.

6.  In the 1960s, several educational organizations were established in response to popular labor coping methods. The methods were *psychoprophylaxis* (the Lamaze method) and *natural* or *husband-coached* childbirth (proposed by Robert Bradley, an obstetrician who advocated substituting special breathing techniques for pharmacologic analgesia). Prominent organizations were the American Society for Psychoprophylaxis in Obstetrics and the American Academy of Husband Coached Childbirth.

 7.  **The term natural childbirth initially described a particular approach to childbirth—labor and birth without analgesia or anesthesia. However, it has come to mean being prepared for the birth experience through information, instruction, exercises, and techniques developed to deal with the discomforts of pregnancy, labor, and birth. Childbirth education has become a standard part of prenatal care in the United States.**

8.  Regardless of the approach, all types of childbirth education classes commonly provide information about prenatal care and planning for the birth, fetal growth and development, preparation for labor and delivery, and postpartum care of the mother and newborn.

 9.  **Inclusion of fathers and other family members in the birthing process is an important aspect of childbirth education.**

10. Because individuals vary in their response to stress and because the characteristics of individual labor vary, the carefully considered use of pain medication along with breathing and relaxation techniques may enhance the woman's ability to maintain control during the labor process.

11. Childbirth educators see themselves as expectant parents' advocates. Childbirth education has grown from a small consumer movement to a significant force in maternity care in the United States.

**B.** **Goals of childbirth education**

1.  Provide expectant parents with knowledge and skills necessary to cope with the stresses of pregnancy, labor, and birth.

2.  Prepare expectant parents to be informed healthcare consumers.

3.  Assist parents in achieving a positive, safe, and rewarding labor and birth experience.

**C.** **Effectiveness of childbirth education**
  1. Learning stress reduction and relaxation techniques, the woman copes more effectively with the stress of labor.
  2. Unsupported claims include improving the spouse's relationship and facilitating painless labor.

  3. **Neonatal health is improved with minimal or no analgesia or anesthesia during labor and birth.**
  4. Parent–newborn bonding is facilitated when mother and newborn are awake and aware at the time of birth.

**D.** **Birth plan**
  1. Some childbearing couples select their primary birthing attendant (eg, obstetrician) and allow the attendant to make decisions on their behalf. Other couples decide what they want in the childbearing experience and choose their primary birthing attendant accordingly.
  2. Decisions to be made by the childbearing couple include:
     a. Determining where they prefer the birth to occur (eg, hospital with traditional maternity center or birthing center, community agency, private hospital, free-standing birthing center, home)
     b. Selecting birthing attendant (eg, obstetrician, pediatrician, family practice physician, midwife)
     c. Selecting a preferred birthing approach and devising a plan
  3. Couples need to understand how birth plans can be modified to meet the specific demands and changes of their birth experience.

## II. Prenatal and postpartum teaching

**A.** **Prenatal education programs**
  1. Programs vary widely in length, goals, and content.
  2. First-trimester classes commonly focus on such issues as early physiologic changes, fetal development, sexuality during pregnancy, and nutrition; some early sessions may include prepregnant couples.
  3. Second- and third-trimester classes may focus on preparation for birth, parenting, and newborn care.

**B.** **Content of childbirth education classes**
  1. Prenatal care and planning
     a. Nutrition, exercise, rest
     b. Parental discomforts and self-care measures
     c. Making a birth plan
     d. Choosing a birth setting, primary care provider, and birth approach
     e. Recognition of danger signs and symptoms

2. Fetal development
   a. Maternal drug and medication use
   b. Maternal nutrition
   c. Environmental hazards
   d. Developmental milestones
3. Preparation for labor and delivery
   a. Muscle toning exercises
   b. Breathing techniques
   c. Relaxation exercises
   d. Analgesia and anesthesia
   e. Preparation for possible cesarean delivery
4. Postpartum care
   a. Self-care
   b. Newborn care
   c. Feeding methods
   d. Maternal nutrition, exercise, and rest needs
   e. Recognition of danger signs and symptoms

C. **Approaches to childbirth education**
   1. Grantly Dick-Read suggests that education decreases fear, tension, and pain; teaches exercises to improve muscle tone and increase relaxation; and stresses slow breathing, muscle relaxation, and pushing techniques.
   2. The Lamaze or psychoprophylactic method combines relaxation, concentration, focusing, and complex, well-paced breathing patterns to reduce the perception of pain through a conditioned response to labor contractions.
   3. The Bradley technique focuses on slow breathing and deep relaxation for labor; reduced responsiveness to external stimuli; and the role of the male partner as coach. It is basically Dick-Read's approach with the addition of a labor coach.
   4. The Wright or "new childbirth" method involves slower but more complex breathing patterns than the Lamaze method.
   5. The Kitzinger method uses sensory memory as an aid to understanding and working with the body in preparation for childbirth.
   6. Yoga teaches relaxation, concentration, and "complete breathing" (combination of chest and abdominal breathing).
   7. Hypnosis may be of benefit for some clients.
    8. **Contemporary childbirth education methods tend to be eclectic, combining features of many approaches, particularly Dick-Read, Lamaze, and Bradley.**

D. **Teaching methods**
   1. Individual teaching and counseling
   2. Groups and classes structured as informational classes, counseling groups, or discussion groups

**E.** Postpartum education programs

    **1.** With the emergence of shorter hospital stays, classes following delivery are being offered through hospitals, clinics, private agencies, and health professionals in private practice.

    **2.** Although these programs vary widely in length, goals, and content, they all provide support for parents.

    **3.** These programs often are extensions of the prenatal classes and deal with issues as they emerge from parents' concerns (eg, mother's body image concerns, fertility and infertility, parenting).

**F.** Sibling preparation classes

 **1.** **Purposes include preparing children for what to expect when they visit mother and newborn in the hospital, reducing the problems associated with separation when mother goes to the hospital, and facilitating the parents' preparation of children for the introduction of the newborn in the home.**

    **2.** Few programs prepare children for attendance at birth; a sibling-support person is usually expected to accompany the child to reduce distraction of mother during labor.

**G.** Grandparent preparation classes

    **1.** Classes are frequently offered in maternity centers that encourage grandparent visits, holding the newborn, and extended visiting hours.

 **2.** **Purposes include increasing grandparents' awareness of changes that have occurred in childbearing and childrearing and increasing grandparents' awareness of their own feelings.**

    **3.** Some grandparents are an integral part of the birthing experience and need information about being a "coach."

    **4.** The need for knowledgeable extended family support systems becomes increasingly important with shorter hospital stays.

**H.** Breast-feeding programs

    **1.** Content includes preparation of breasts, techniques for breast-feeding, and advantages versus disadvantages of breast-feeding (Table 7-1).

    **2.** These classes are offered by hospitals, birthing centers, clinics, individuals, and the La Leche League.

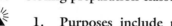 **3.** **Fathers are included more frequently, because these programs provide an opportunity to express their feelings—both positive and negative—about breast-feeding.**

TABLE 7–1.

Comparing Features of Breast-feeding and Bottle Feeding

| FEATURES | BREAST-FEEDING | BOTTLE FEEDING |
|---|---|---|
| **Advantages** | ▶ Breast milk is considered ideal food source for newborn.<br>▶ No special preparations or supplies are needed.<br>▶ Breast-feeding speeds involution (return of uterus to normal size) for mother.<br>▶ Maternal antibodies transferred in breast milk decrease incidence of allergies. | ▶ Feeding preparation replicates mother's milk as nearly as possible.<br>▶ Formula containers are marked, making it easy to measure newborn's intake.<br>▶ Father can participate in feeding and bonding.<br>▶ Immediately replenishable supply of formula helps to satisfy appetite of larger newborns. |
| **Disadvantages** | ▶ It takes about 3 weeks for milk supply and breast to become fully established during which time a large newborn may be unsatisfied.<br>▶ It may be inconvenient or difficult for mother employed outside of home.<br>▶ Physical and psychological preparations for breast-feeding may be too demanding or inconvenient for some women.<br>▶ Father cannot participate in feeding newborn. | ▶ Some feeding formulas may contribute to colic.<br>▶ Feeding formula does not contain immune bodies from mother.<br>▶ Feeding formula may require extensive preparation (supplies, measuring, mixing, storage).<br>▶ Method requires planning; parents must pack and carry feeding supplies when away from home.<br>▶ Bottle feeding costs more than breast-feeding.<br>▶ Preparation of formula increases chance for feeding error. |

## III. Implications for nursing management
### A. Assessment
1. Determine the woman's or couple's expectations about instruction and about childbirth.
2. Evaluate clients' knowledge of:
   a. Anatomy and physiology of pregnancy
   b. Fetal development
   c. What to expect during prenatal visits
   d. Preparation for labor and delivery
   e. Newborn care
   f. Self-care
### B. Nursing diagnoses
1. Anxiety
2. Fear
3. Knowledge Deficit
4. Ineffective Management of Therapeutic Regimen: Noncompliance
5. Powerlessness

**C. Planning and implementation**

1. Use standard adult-learning principles in childbirth education.
2. Alleviate anxiety and fear and promote client control by maintaining an open nonjudgmental atmosphere.
3. Address client questions and concerns honestly and promptly to help boost compliance with the program.
4. After assessing individual or group needs, plan instruction as appropriate on such topics as:
   a. Minor discomforts and their alleviation
   b. Fetal growth and development
   c. Nutritional needs during pregnancy and lactation
   d. Newborn care, such as sleeping and waking patterns, newborn safety, bathing and feeding techniques, cord care, circumcision
   e. Prenatal assessment and diagnostic testing of fetal status (eg, complete blood profile, urinalysis, and routine ultrasonography, with at-risk clients possibly undergoing maternal–fetal activity assessment, estriol determinations, non-stress test, contraction stress test, or amniocentesis)
   f. **Danger signs and symptoms (eg, spotting, headaches, edema, unusual pain, increased temperature, painful urination, signs of preterm labor); client to report these at once**
   g. Preparation for labor and delivery (eg, signs and symptoms of true labor, when to go to the hospital or call the physician or midwife, plans for getting to the hospital with alternate options, understanding the admission process, what to expect of medical and nursing care, fetal monitoring techniques and purpose, breathing techniques during labor, relaxation techniques between contractions, analgesia during labor and delivery, hydration during labor)
   h. Preparation for feeding, including advantages and disadvantages of breast-feeding and bottle feeding.
   i. Preparation for analgesia and anesthesia during labor and delivery, including advantages and disadvantages of available options: natural childbirth, regional anesthesia, systemic medications, inhalation anesthesia, general anesthesia
   j. Sibling preparation for birth, including:
      ▶ Involvement of children during antepartum period and labor and delivery (eg, listening to fetal heart tones, feeling fetal movements and kicking, naming the newborn, doll play)
      ▶ Intrapartal visitation, advantages and disadvantages, preparation for holding the newborn

       ► Postpartum sibling visits, early discharge of mother, sibling involvement in helping mother
       ► Expecting and coping with sibling rivalry (eg, providing extra attention, giving siblings undivided attention before introducing newborn to them)

  k.  Grandparent preparation for birth, including:

       ► Community support classes
       ► Discussions on how to provide help without "smothering" parents (eg, when to babysit)
       ► Involvement during labor and delivery

  l.  Preparation for possible cesarean birth, including indications, advantages and disadvantages, risks, partner's involvement, anesthesia

**5.  Integrate the father into preparation for childbirth. Provide such information as:**
  a.  **How to coach the mother during labor and delivery**
  b.  **The importance of helping partner keep antenatum appointments**
  c.  **The significance of fetal heart tones (FHTs) and the sonogram; listening to FHTs and viewing the sonogram**
  d.  **How he can participate in preparing the home for the newborn**
  e.  **Preparing siblings for the newborn**

**D.  Evaluation**
  1.  The expectant parents verbalize decreased anxiety and fear related to pregnancy and childbirth.
  2.  The expectant parents voice a feeling of control in planning for delivery and choosing a primary caregiver.
  3.  The parents demonstrate understanding of the assessments and diagnostic tests done during pregnancy.
  4.  Parents participate in childbirth education process.
  5.  The father verbalizes an understanding of his role in the childbirth process.
  6.  The couple verbalizes an understanding of the major concepts and content of childbirth education classes.
  7.  The parents are able to discuss with the primary caregiver the options for analgesia and anesthesia.
  8.  The parents state the circumstances that may necessitate a cesarean birth.
  9.  The parents verbalize danger signs and the need to report them promptly.
  10.  The parents explore various feeding methods.

11. The mother verbalizes important aspects of newborn care and self-care in the postpartum period.

## Bibliography

Bobak, I. M., & Jensen, M. D. (1993). *Maternity and gynecologic care: The nurse and the family* (5th ed.). St. Louis: C.V. Mosby.

Gorrie, T. M., McKinney, E. S., & Murray, S. S. (1994). *Foundations of maternal newborn nursing*. Philadelphia: W.B. Saunders.

May, K. A., & Mahlmeister, L. R. (1994). *Maternal and neonatal nursing: Family-centered care* (3rd ed.). Philadelphia: J.B. Lippincott.

McElmurry, B. J., & Parker, R. S. (Ed.) (1993). *Annual review of women's health*. New York: National League for Nursing.

Olds, S. B., London, M. L., & Ladewig, P. W. (1992). *Maternal-newborn nursing: A family centered approach* (4th ed.). Menlo Park, CA: Addison-Wesley.

Reeder, S. J., Martin, L. L., & Koniak, D. (1992). *Maternity nursing: Family newborn, and women's health care* (17th ed.). Philadelphia: J.B. Lippincott.

## STUDY QUESTIONS

1. The first formal childbirth education classes in the United States were offered by which of the following?
   a. The English physician, Grantly Dick-Read
   b. The International Childbirth Education Association
   c. The American Red Cross
   d. The American Society for Psychoprophylaxis in Obstetrics

2. Select the best definition of childbirth education.
   a. It is the standard part of prenatal care in this country as advocated by Grantly Dick-Read.
   b. It is the most popular prenatal program because it advocates "natural childbirth" without analgesia and advocates coaching.
   c. It assists parents in achieving a positive, safe, and rewarding labor and birth experience.
   d. It describes the information, exercises, and techniques developed and used to deal with the discomforts of pregnancy, labor, and birth.

3. In which period of pregnancy would the focus of classes be mainly on physiologic changes, fetal development, sexuality during pregnancy, and nutrition?
   a. During the first trimester
   b. During the prepregnant period
   c. During the second trimester
   d. During the third trimester

4. Which of the following approaches to childbirth education advocates slow breathing, deep relaxation, and a person to act as coach?
   a. The Dick-Read method
   b. The "new childbirth" method
   c. The Bradley method
   d. The Lamaze method

5. From the following, select the best purpose for sibling preparation classes:
   a. They prepare the child for what to expect when visiting mother during labor and delivery.
   b. They prepare the child to visit mother and newborn in the hospital and for babysitting when at home.
   c. They prepare the child for what to expect when visiting mother and newborn in the hospital.
   d. They prepare the child to understand the important reasons why mother cannot give him or her all of the attention.

6. From the following, select the best purpose for grandparent preparation classes:
   a. They help prepare the grandparents for hospital visits during labor and delivery.
   b. They help to increase the grandparents' awareness of changes that have occurred in childbearing.
   c. They help to prepare the grandparents to be more up to date in babysitting situations.
   d. They help prepare the grandparents for the emotional problems of aging and becoming grandparents.

7. From the following groups of signs and symptoms, select the group considered to be dangerous during pregnancy:
   a. Spotting, headaches, edema, unusual pain, and increased temperature
   b. Spotting, headaches, constipation, increased fever, and cramping
   c. Constipation, painful urination, increased fever, and headaches
   d. Cramping, back pain, increased temperature, headaches, and edema

8. Breast-feeding has several advantages and disadvantages. Which of the following would be one of the disadvantages?
   a. Involution occurs more rapidly, and breast milk contains immune bodies.
   b. It is considered the best food for the newborn and costs less.
   c. The father cannot feed or bond as well.

d. There is less chance of error during preparation.

9. From the following, select the best reason for a father to be included in breast-feeding programs:
   a. He will be able to understand why his wife has to spend so much time with the newborn.
   b. He will be prepared to explain the procedure of breast-feeding to the other children at home.
   c. He will be able to help his wife with problems of self-esteem, body image, and frustration.
   d. He will have an opportunity to express his feelings—both positive and negative—about breast-feeding.

10. Which of the following best describes the effectiveness of childbirth education?
    a. It provides expectant parents with knowledge and skills necessary to cope with pregnancy.
    b. It prepares expectant parents to be informed consumers of birthing attendants and facilities.
    c. It provides a long time for expectant parents to express their concerns and fears.
    d. It improves newborn health, parent–newborn bonding, and helps the woman to cope with labor.

---

For additional questions, see
*Lippincott's Self-Study Series* Software
Available at your bookstore

# ANSWER KEY

94

**1. Correct response: c**
The first formal childbirth education classes in the United States were offered by the American Red Cross in 1913 as a result of concern for public health.
  **a, b, and d.** All of these contributed to childbirth education but came after 1913.
*Knowledge/Health Promotion/NA*

**2. Correct response: d**
It describes the information, exercises, and techniques used to deal with the discomforts of pregnancy, labor, and birth.
  **a, b, and c.** These are not definitions of childbirth education.
*Knowledge/Health Promotion/
Implementation*

**3. Correct response: a**
First-trimester classes commonly focus on such issues as early physiologic changes, fetal development, sexuality during pregnancy, and nutrition; some early classes may include prepregnant couples.
  **b, c, and d.** Second- and third-trimester classes may focus on preparation for birth, parenting, and newborn care.
*Application/Health Promotion/
Implementation*

**4. Correct response: c**
The Bradley technique focuses on slow breathing and deep relaxation for labor, reduced responsiveness to external stimuli, and the role for an individual as a coach; it is basically Dick-Read's approach with the addition of a labor coach.
  **a, b, and d.** All are incorrect.
*Application/Health Promotion/
Implementation*

**5. Correct response: c**
They prepare the child for what to ex-pect when visiting mother and newborn in the hospital.
  **a.** There are few programs that prepare the child for attendance at birth; a sibling support person is usually expected to accompany the child to reduce distraction of mother during labor.
  **b and d.** These are incorrect.
*Knowledge/Health Promotion/
Implementation*

**6. Correct response: b**
They help to increase the grandparents' awareness of changes that have occurred in childbearing.
  **a, c, and d.** These are incorrect.
*Knowledge/Health Promotion/
Implementation*

**7. Correct response: a**
Together, spotting, headaches, edema, unusual pain, and increased temperature are dangerous.
  **b, c, and d.** All may appear at times, but not all of them are danger signs and symptoms.
*Application/Health Promotion/
Implementation*

**8. Correct response: c**
The father cannot feed the newborn and therefore may have more difficulty or may have fewer chances for bonding.
  **a, b, and d.** All are advantages of breast-feeding.
*Analysis/Health Promotion/
Implementation*

**9. Correct response: d**
Fathers are included more frequently because these programs provide an opportunity for expression of their feelings—both positive and negative—about breast-feeding.
  **a, b, and c.** These are incorrect answers.
*Analysis/Health Promotion/
Implementation*

**10.** *Correct response: d*
It improves newborn health and parent–newborn bonding and helps the woman cope with labor.

**a and b.** These are goals of childbirth education.
**c.** This is incorrect.
*Knowledge/Health Promotion/Implementation*

# Antepartum Care

## I. Overview

### A. Essential concepts

1. **Antepartum care refers to the medical and nursing care given to the pregnant woman between conception and the onset of labor.**

2. Consideration is given to the physical, emotional, and social needs of the woman, the unborn child, her partner, and other family members.

3. **Pregnancy is viewed as a normal physiologic process, not a disease process.** Nevertheless, at no other time in life does a woman need such intense, regular care as during pregnancy.

4. With the advent of highly sophisticated instrumentation and monitoring, the nurse must be particularly alert that these techniques are used to augment practice and should never replace the therapeutic process.

 **5. Although the value of prenatal care in terms of maternal-fetal outcome is well documented, prenatal care—even of the highest quality—does not guarantee a positive outcome.**

6. The process of data gathering and analysis is ongoing; the nurse cannot expect to cover all areas during the initial antepartum visit and therefore should focus on trimester-specific issues.

7. Every woman who has been menstruating and who misses a menstrual period is usually considered pregnant until proven otherwise. Pregnancy must be ruled out in any instance of amenorrhea, even though the woman insists that she is not pregnant.

8. The following methods are commonly used to determine pregnancy:
   a. Pregnancy tests (urine or serum) at home or in the health care facility
   b. presumptive evidence of pregnancy (amenorrhea, nausea, breast tenderness)
   c. probable evidence of pregnancy (enlarged abdomen, quickening)
   d. positive evidence of pregnancy (fetal heart beat, ultrasound visualization)

9. Pregnancy tests are not infallible. A negative result may occur when pregnancy exists or a positive result when there is no pregnancy (Table 8-1).

**B. Expected outcomes of antepartum care**
1. The expectant mother's and family's knowledge of pregnancy increases.
2. The expectant mother and other family members learn about actions they can take to facilitate a positive birth outcome.
3. Family members experience pregnancy in a positive way.
4. The newborn is successfully integrated into the family.

**C. Factors affecting the antepartum experience**
1. Previous experience with pregnancy
2. Cultural and personal expectations
3. Prepregnant health and biophysical preparedness for childbearing
4. Motivation for childbearing
5. Socioeconomic status
6. Mother's age and partnered versus unpartnered status

TABLE 8–1.
Causes of False Pregnancy Test Results

| CAUSES | FALSE-POSITIVES | FALSE-NEGATIVES |
|---|---|---|
| Human | Error in reading<br>Error in recording | Error in reading<br>Error in recording |
| Poor test sample or condition | Recent pregnancy (eg, test done fewer than 10 days after abortion)<br>Proteinuria<br>Hematuria<br>Test performed during ovulation | Test performed too early or too late in pregnancy<br>Urine too dilute<br>Urine stored too long at room temperature |
| Substance interference | Luteinizing hormone cross-reaction (as in menopause)<br>Aspirin in large doses, phenothiazines (antipsychotic medications), marijuana, methyldopa (Aldomet)<br>Treatment with human chorionic gonadotropin (HCG) for infertility (affects blood tests only)<br>HCG secreted by tumor | N/A |
| Other | Pregnancy recently terminated (within 10 days of test)<br>Trophoblastic disease (molar pregnancy or choriocarcinoma) | Missed abortion<br>Ectopic pregnancy<br>Impending spontaneous abortion |

      7.   Accessibility of prenatal care

      8.   Level of education

  **D.**  **Nursing responsibilities**

      1.   **Perform trimester-specific physiologic and psychosocial assessment, and facilitate follow-up care as needed.**

      2.   Provide education and counseling for the pregnant woman and her family.

      3.   Make appropriate referrals for additional services as needed.

**II.**  **Essentials of antepartum assessment**

  **A.**  **Health history**

      1.   Current pregnancy: first day of last menstrual period, cramping or bleeding, results of pregnancy test, discomfort (eg, nausea, vomiting, headache, urinary frequency, fatigue)

      2.   History of previous pregnancies: gravida, para, number of abortions, number of living children, prenatal education, cesarean births

      3.   Gynecologic history: previous infections; previous surgery, age of menarche and menstrual cycle; sexual, menstrual, and contraception history

      4.   Current medical history: weight, blood type and Rh, medica-

tions presently taking (prescription and over the counter), habits (smoking, alcohol, caffeine, drugs), allergies, potential teratogenic effects on this pregnancy (eg, infections, medications, radiographs, toxins in home or workplace), medical conditions (diabetes, hypertension, cardiovascular, renal, congenital), immunizations

5. Medical history: childhood diseases, medical diseases and treatment, sexually transmitted diseases, surgeries, bleeding disorders or previous blood transfusions, emotional problems, accidents

6. Family medical history: medical disorders (eg, cancer, heart disease, diabetes), multiple births, genetic or congenital disorders

7. Occupational history: type of work and health hazards

8. History of baby's father: age, health problems, habits, blood type and Rh, genetic or congenital disorders, occupation, attitude toward pregnancy

9. Personal information: racial, cultural, and religious practices; exercise; housing and living conditions; income; support system; use of health care system; work

**B. Assessment of risk factors**

1. Early identification of potential risk factors may provide opportunities for appropriate interventions.

2. Risk factors that could have a negative effect on the pregnancy may be characterized as demographic, obstetric, medical, and miscellaneous (Table 8-2).

**C. Diagnostic tests and procedures**

1. During the initial assessment of physical status, which typically occurs during the first prenatal visits, baseline data are obtained, providing a measure against which subsequent data are evaluated.

2. Laboratory tests include:
   a. Urine tests: protein, glucose, ketones, bilirubin, blood, white blood cells, bacteria
   b. Blood tests: hemoglobin and hematocrit; *blood type, Rh, and antibody titer; rubella screen*; serology; hemoglobin electrophoresis; *hepatitis B; human immunodeficiency virus* testing; sickle cell screen
   c. Diabetes screen: usually done at 24 to 28 weeks' gestation because of hormonal effects that block insulin usage
   d. Cultures: Pap, gonorrhea, vaginal smear

**III. Evaluation of fetal well-being**

**A. Essential concepts**

1. Maternal weight gain, uterine growth, fetal activity, and fetal heart rate (FHR) are usually assessed at each prenatal visit.

TABLE 8–2.
Perinatal Risk Assessment

| AREAS TO BE ASSESSED | CONDITIONS ASSOCIATED WITH INCREASED RISK |
|---|---|

**Antepartum Course**

General prenatal information

Lack of prenatal care
Weight gain ≤ 15 lb or ≥ 35 lb

Maternal health

Medical conditions:
   Insulin-dependent diabetes*
   Heart disease
   Chronic hypertension
Habits
   Smoking
   Substance abuse
Infections during pregnancy:
   Rubella
   Veneral disease
Complications of pregnancy:
   Pregnancy-induced hypertension
   Third-trimester bleeding*
   Rh sensitization; severe sensitization*
   Multiple fetuses*

Results of antepartum tests

Estriol levels: ↓ or no ↑ after 36 wk
Ultrasound: growth retardation ≥2 wk
Amniocentesis:
   Bilirubin or meconium present
   L/S ratio <2:1
Nonstress test: nonreactive
Stress test: positive

**Intrapartum Course**

Length of pregnancy

<34 wk, ≤37 wk, ≥42 wk
Prolonged first or second stage*

Duration and character of labor

Precipitous labor or delivery
Premature rupture of membrane > 24 h
Difficult labor
Cephalopelvic disproportion

Maternal conditions

Preexisting problems (see antepartum course)
Progressive hypotension
Progressive hypertension
Excessive bleeding*
Signs of Infection
   Severe*

Fetal presentation and position

Breech*
Transverse lie*

Events indicating possible fetal distress

Fetal monitoring findings
   Persistent late decelerations*
   Severe variable decelerations*
   Heart rate < 120 or > 160 for > 30 min
   Poor beat-to-beat (short-term and long-term) variability
Scalp pH ≤ 7.25*

(continued)

TABLE 8–2. (continued)

| AREAS TO BE ASSESSED | CONDITIONS ASSOCIATED WITH INCREASED RISK |
| --- | --- |
| | Meconium-stained fluid* |
| | Prolapsed cord* |
| Analgesia | Large or repeated doses of analgesia (eg, meperidine may cause neonatal respiratory depression for up to 4 h after administration) |
| | IM analgesia between 1 and 4 h of delivery |
| | IV analgesia within 1/2 h of delivery |
| Anesthesia | General anesthesia |
| | Conduction anesthesia with maternal hypotension |
| Method of delivery | Cesarean delivery* |
| | Midforceps or high-forceps delivery* |
| | Failed vacuum extraction |

*Conditions usually requiring presence at delivery of someone skilled in resuscitation.*

2. In approximately 20% of pregnancies, further assessment of fetal well-being is indicated.
3. First-trimester fetal assessments typically include auscultation of FHR and ultrasonography.
4. Second-trimester assessments typically include measurements of fundal height, FHR, fetal movement (quickening), and ultrasonography.
5. Third-trimester assessment includes monitoring fetal movement and ultrasonography.

**B. FHR**

1. FHR usually is auscultated at the midline suprapubic region with a Doppler ultrasound stethoscope at 10 to 12 weeks' gestation.
2. FHR can be auscultated with a fetoscope at about 20 weeks' gestation.

3. **An FHR of 120 to 160 beats/min can be distinguished from the slower maternal heart rate by palpating the mother's pulse while auscultating the FHR.**
4. FHR is determined at each visit.
5. A regular heart beat is normal; irregularity is abnormal.
6. The heart beat will be muffled when the mother's abdominal wall is thick, if she is obese, or if there is a large volume of amniotic fluid.
7. Fundic souffle, caused by blood rushing through the umbilical arteries, is synchronous with the FHR; uterine souffle, the sound of blood passing through the uterine blood vessels, is synchronous with the maternal pulse.

8.  **Failure to hear FHR may result from inexperience with fetoscope, defective fetoscope or a noisy environment, early pregnancy and small-for-gestational-age fetus, fetal death, obesity, hydramnios, loud placental souffle obscuring the FHR, and posterior position of the fetus.**

C.  **Ultrasonography (sonograms)**

   1.  Serial sonograms provide useful information when assessing fetal growth and well-being.

   2.  Ultrasonography provides different information during different trimesters:

      a.  First trimester

         ► Assessment of gestational age
         ► Evaluation for congenital anomalies
         ► Diagnostic evaluation of vaginal bleeding
         ► Confirmation of suspected multiple gestation
         ► Evaluation of fetal growth
         ► Adjunct to prenatal testing (amniocentesis, chorionic villus sampling)
         ► Diagnostic evaluation of pelvic mass

      b.  Second trimester

         ► Assessment of gestational age
         ► Evaluation of congenital anomalies (eg, hydrocephaly)
         ► Assessment of fetal growth
         ► Guidance of procedures, such as amniocentesis and fetoscopy
         ► Assessment of placental location
         ► Diagnosis of multiple gestation

      c.  Third trimester

         ► Determination of fetal position
         ► Estimation of fetal size

   3.  **Second-trimester sonogram is recommended as a baseline for all clients considered to be at risk for complications.**

   4.  A full bladder may improve ultrasonic resolution before 20 weeks' gestation. During the first trimester, clients may be instructed to drink a quart or more of fluid 1 to 2 hours before the procedure.

   5.  When used as an adjunct to prenatal diagnoses, ultrasonic visualization of the fetus may contribute to the difficulty of pregnancy termination decisions.

   6.  It is possible to visualize the head, extremities, moving heart valves and frequently the sex of the fetus. The parents should be asked whether they want to know the sex of the child before providing this information.

**D.** **Measurement of fundal height**

    1.    Assessment begins during the second trimester when the fundus is palpable until the end of pregnancy.

    2.    McDonald's measurement involves using a nonelastic but flexible measuring tape, placing the zero point on the superior border of the symphysis pubis, and stretching the tape across the abdomen at the midline to the top of the fundus.

    **3.**    **After 20 to 22 weeks' gestation, the fundal height in centimeters normally approximates the gestational age in weeks until after the 36th week.**

    4.    Possible causes of greater-than-expected fundal height include multiple gestation, polyhydramnios, and fetal macrosomia.

    5.    Possible causes for less-than-expected fundal height include abnormal fetal presentation, fetal growth retardation, congenital anomalies, and oligohydramnios.

**E.** **Fetal movement (quickening)**

    1.    In primigravidas (first-time mothers), quickening normally is detected between 18 and 20 weeks' gestation.

    2.    In secundigravidas and multigravidas, quickening may occur as early as 16 weeks.

    3.    Quickening is typically described as a light fluttering feeling; it may be mistaken for flatus.

**F.** **Electronic fetal heart monitoring (EFHM)**

    1.    EFHM is used during the antepartum period to evaluate a high-risk fetus.

    2.    It demonstrates fetal heart response to spontaneous or induced uterine contractions.

    3.    Contractions stress the fetus by decreasing uterine perfusion. In a fetus already compromised by disease, cord compression, or other factors, contractions may alter heart rate, which is detectable on EFHM.

    4.    Common EFHM studies include the nonstress test (NST) and the contraction stress test (CST).

    5.    NST

        a.    This is the least invasive test of fetal well-being, involving the use of an electronic fetal monitor. The baseline FHR and the presence of periodic patterns are identified and correlated to contractions observed on the uterine activity tracing.

        b.    Adequate perfusion is necessary to maintain fetal central nervous system integrity and reflex responses.

        c.    In a healthy fetus, fetal movement causes an accelerated heart rate; in this case, the test is reactive.

        d.    Among the various assessment protocols, the most common involves two FHR accelerations within a 10-minute period, with each acceleration increasing heart rate by at least 15 beats/min and lasting at least 15 seconds.

 e. **The fetus typically is monitored for at least 40 minutes (to account for a normal sleep period); the entire tracing is then evaluated.**

f. Abnormal or nonreactive NST results require further evaluation that same day.

g. Even with a reactive NST, follow-up is indicated if FHR falls outside the range of 120 to 160 beats/min or if decelerations (early, late, or variable) are detected.

6. CST

a. Perfusion through the spinal arteries of the uterus decreases during contractions. Recordings of the heart rate of the fetus with limited reserve show late decelerations in response to the stress of contractions (a positive CST finding). The healthy fetus responds to the stress of contractions with a normal heart rate and no decelerations apparent on the fetal monitoring strip (a negative CST result).

b. During fetal testing, contractions may occur spontaneously; most often, however, stimulation will be necessary. This is done either by breast stimulation (eg, nipple rolling or application of moist hot pads) to trigger prolactin release or by low-dose oxytocin infusion (oxytocin challenge test [OCT]).

c. Three contractions within 10 minutes—ideally, lasting 40 to 60 seconds each—must be evaluated to assess fetal response to stress.

d. **During an OCT, oxytocin may precipitate labor.**

G. **Other procedures**

1. Amniocentesis can determine fetal maturity and detect certain birth defects (eg, Down syndrome, spina bifida), hemolytic disease of the newborn, and sex and chromosomal abnormalities.

2. Chorionic villus biopsy is done early in pregnancy to detect fetal abnormalities.

3. Routine maternal urine and serum assays help monitor fetal status. In serum, for example, human chorionic gonadotropin indicates a viable fetus, estriol and human placental lactogen reflect fetal homeostasis.

4. Fetoscopy enables direct fetal visualization through a fetoscope, an optical instrument, inserted through the abdominal and uterine walls to identify developmental abnormalities. The

fetoscope also can retrieve tissue and blood samples to detect hemophilia or other disorders.

5. Amnioscopy (transcervical fetal visualization) and radiographs are less common.

6. Percutaneous umbilical blood sampling (Fig. 8-1), also called cordocentesis, may be performed in the second or third trimesters to investigate or treat conditions requiring direct access to the fetal vascular system.

## IV. Implications for nursing management

### A. Initial assessment

1. Vital signs, height, and weight (current and prepregnant)
2. Systematic, thorough physical examination, including pelvic examination
3. Determination of estimated date of delivery (EDD) or estimated date of confinement

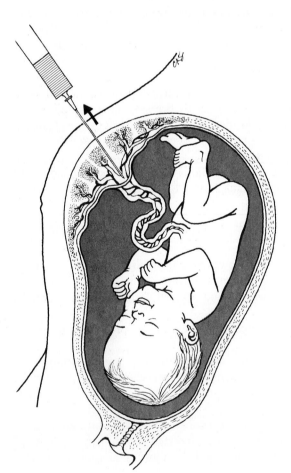

FIGURE 8–1.
Percutaneous umbilical blood sampling involves inserting a needle into the fetal umbilical cord and aspirating blood for analysis. The procedure is guided by ultrasonography and is used to screen karyotypes (chromosomes), examine antibodies for teratogenic viruses, and provide access for fetal blood transfusions.

a. **The average length of pregnancy is 280 days (40 weeks, 10 lunar months, or 9 calendar months), as calculated from the first day of the last menstrual period (LMP)**

b. To calculate the EDD by Nägele's rule, determine the LMP. Add 7 days to the first day of the LMP, and count back 3 months to arrive at the EDD.

c. Dating pregnancy when LMP is unknown:

▸ Uterine size is reported in terms of weeks of gestation at the first prenatal visit.

▸ Presence of the uterus in the abdomen (fundal height) indicates at least 12 weeks' gestation.

▸ Uterus in the pelvis (fundal height) indicates less than 12 weeks' gestation.

▸ Quickening indicates about 20 weeks' gestation in primigravidas; fewer in multigravidas.

▸ Fetal heart tones can be detected at 10 to 12 weeks' gestation with Doppler ultrasound and at 16 to 20 weeks with a fetoscope.

▸ Ultrasound can detect pregnancy 5 to 6 weeks after last menstrual period.

4. Assessment of pelvic size for adequacy (See Chap. 2 for discussion of pelvic measurements.):

a. Measurement of the dimensions and proportion of the bony pelvis

b. Obtained during bimanual portion of the pelvic examination by moving the fingers over the landmarks of the bony pelvis and estimating their size

c. May be delayed until later in pregnancy when the procedure may be more comfortable for the mother, because it is not crucial to determine pelvic adequacy at the initial assessment

5. Inspection and palpation of breasts for normal and questionable changes of pregnancy

a. Normal changes associated with pregnancy: increased size, tenderness, darkening and enlargement of areola, erection of nipples and leaking of colostrum late in first trimester, appearance of venous pattern and striae formation

b. Questionable changes: recent lumps or masses that feel hard or fixed, dimpling, redness, edema, ulceration, nipple retraction or elevation

6. Psychosocial assessment during initial visit(s):

a. Determining expectations for pregnancy, emotional and

financial impact on family, partner's attitude toward pregnancy (eg, excitement or apprehension)

b. Whether or not the pregnancy was planned

c. Educational needs and resources

d. Support systems

e. Religious beliefs and cultural practices related to childbirth and parenting

f. Family functioning, living situation, sexual activity

g. Preparation for parenthood; preparation for childbirth

**B. Subsequent prenatal visit assessments**

1. **Frequency of prenatal visits: every 4 weeks for the first 28 weeks; every 2 weeks from 28 to 36 weeks; then weekly until delivery**

2. Physical assessment with each prenatal visit:

   a. Data concerning course of pregnancy (eg, common discomforts and how alleviated)

   b. Maternal vital signs: temperature, pulse, respiration, and blood pressure

   c. Weight gain (distribution per trimester)

   d. Presence of edema

   e. Uterine size (ballottement and engagement)

   f. FHR

   g. Urine for protein and glucose

    h. **Danger signals: vaginal bleeding, blurred vision, leaking of amniotic fluid, rapid weight gain, elevated blood pressure**

   i. After 38 weeks, signs of impending labor: lightening, engagement, cervical status

3. Laboratory tests:

   a. Urine dipstick analysis for glucose, protein, ketones at each visit

   b. Complete blood count or Hgb, hematocrit at each trimester

   c. Rh antibody screen at 24 to 28 weeks if negative or previous sensitization

   d. Sexually transmitted disease tests repeated if indicated

   e. Blood glucose screen at 24 to 28 weeks

4. Educational needs relative to sexual activity, preparation for parenting, preparation for childbirth, knowledge of signs of labor

5. Psychological and emotional status; expression of client's or couple's concerns

6. Nutritional assessment:

   a. Review of dietary intake of iron, iron supplements

    b.    24-hour diet recall

    c.    Comparison of prepregnancy weight with weight gained during pregnancy (During the course of the pregnancy, a total weight gain of 24–30 lb is recommended.)

     **d.**    **Pattern of weight gain: normal—1.5 lb in the first 10 weeks; 9 lb at 20 weeks; 19 lb by 30 weeks; and 27.5 lb by 40 weeks**

    e.    Nondietary factors affecting weight gain (eg, increased blood pressure and excess fluid retention)

**C.** **Assessment of common minor discomforts of pregnancy**

    **1.**    First trimester

        a.    Nausea and vomiting (morning sickness): generally occur after first missed menstrual period and subsides by the fourth month of pregnancy; due to change in hormone levels

        b.    Nasal stuffiness and epistaxis: due to nasal edema from elevated estrogen levels

        c.    Urinary frequency: caused by growing uterus pressing on bladder; seen in first trimester and again in the later part of the third trimester

        d.    Breast tenderness: early in pregnancy, continuing throughout due to hormonal change

        e.    Ptyalism (excessive salvation)

        f.    Leukorrhea (increased vaginal discharge)

        g.    Headaches: due to emotional tension, eye strains, vascular engorgement, and congestion of sinuses from hormonal stimulation

    **2.**    Second and third trimesters

        a.    Heartburn due to regurgitation of acidic gastric contents into the esophagus; may be associated with tension and vomiting in the third trimester

        b.    Ankle edema due to decreased venous return in the lower extremities

        c.    Varicose veins due to poor circulation and weakened vessel walls

        d.    Hemorrhoids due to pressure of the gravid uterus on the spine, which interferes with venous circulation

        e.    Constipation due to decreased intestinal peristalsis and displacement of intestines from a gravid uterus, insufficient fluid intake, or use of iron supplements

        f.    Backache resulting from altered posture due to increased curvature of the lumbosacral vertebrae from the enlarging uterus

        g.    Leg cramps caused by spasms of the gastrocnemius muscle, possibly from insufficient calcium

h.  Faintness due to changes in blood volume and postural hypotension

i.  Shortness of breath due to pressure exerted on the diaphragm by an enlarging uterus

j.  Difficulty sleeping due to an enlarged uterus

 k.  **Round ligament pain due to stretching and hypertrophy of the ligaments; not to be mistaken for labor**

**D.  Nursing diagnoses**

1.  Anxiety
2.  Body Image Disturbance
3.  Altered Bowel Elimination
4.  Family Coping: Potential for Growth
5.  Fear
6.  Health Seeking Behaviors
7.  Knowledge Deficit
8.  Altered Nutrition: Less than body requirements
9.  Altered Nutrition: More than body requirements
10.  Altered Role Performance
11.  Altered Sexuality Patterns
12.  Sexual Dysfunction

**E.  Planning and implementation: first trimester**

1.  Maintain adequate nutritional status. Stress well-balanced meals; review the United States Department of Agriculture's food pyramid, and discuss vitamin and mineral supplementation (Fig. 8-2).

2.  Increase fluid intake to prevent urinary tract infection and improve kidney function.

3.  **Intervene to relieve common discomforts:**

    a.  **Nausea: Instruct client to eat small, dry, bland meals, taking fluids between meals; encourage a snack of dry crackers before arising.**

    b.  **Tiredness: Instruct client to rest whenever possible, get at least 8 hours of sleep each night, and elevate legs when sitting.**

    c.  **Nasal stuffiness: Instruct client to use a cool air vaporizer or humidifier, increase fluid intake, place moist towel on sinuses, and massage sinuses.**

    d.  **Urinary frequency: Encourage client to void when urge is felt and decrease fluid intake in evening.**

    e.  **Breast tenderness: Advise client to wear a supportive bra.**

    f.  **Ptyalism: Encourage use of mouthwash, chewing gum, or sucking on hard candy.**

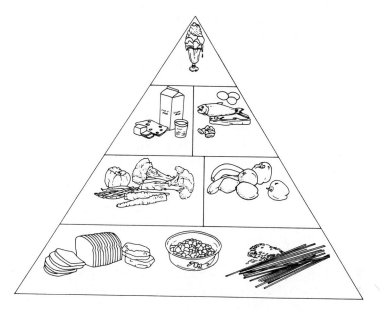

**FIGURE 8–2.**
Food pyramid. In 1992, the United States Department of Agriculture published recommended dietary guidelines. The USDA recommended daily servings from the basic food group of bread, cereal, rice, and pasta (6–11 servings); vegetables (3–5 servings); fruits (2–4 servings); milk, yogurt, and cheese (2–3 servings); meat poultry, fish, dry beans, eggs, and nuts (2–3 servings); and fats and sweets (sparingly). Some single serving equivalents are 1 oz of breakfast cereal, 4 oz of cooked green beans, 2 oz of meat, 1 banana, and 8 oz milk. During pregnancy, recommended daily servings may increase.

      g.   **Leukorrhea: Instruct client to bathe daily, avoid douching, and wear cotton underpants.**

      h.   **Headaches: Instruct client to get enough sleep and rest; eat regular meals; drink fluids; apply cool washcloth to head and back of neck; massage neck, shoulders, face, scalp, and forehead; take warm bath; and relax and meditate.**

   **4.**   Discuss sexual concerns with the client and partner as appropriate; include reasons for altered libido (increased or decreased).

**F.**  **Planning and implementation: second and third trimesters**

   **1.**   Continue to address nutritional needs; assess for normal weight gain.

   **2.**   Intervene for common discomforts:

      a.   Heartburn: Encourage client to eat small, frequent meals and to avoid overeating and spicy, fatty, and fried foods.

      b.   Ankle edema: Instruct client to elevate legs when resting, and caution against wearing tight garters on legs.

     c.    Varicose veins: Instruct client to elevate legs, wear sup-portive hose, and avoid garters, crossing legs, or standing for long periods.

     d.    Hemorrhoids: Encourage regulation of bowel habit with use of stool softener, cold packs or sitz baths, glycerine suppositories, and gentle reinsertion of hemorrhoid with clean, gloved, lubricated finger. Recommend a diet with adequate roughage.

     e.    Constipation: Discuss the importance of adequate dietary fiber intake, increased fluid intake, and exercise; allow use of milk of magnesia, but avoid strong laxatives.

     f.    Backache: Encourage client to maintain good posture and to do the pelvic tilt exercise; encourage client to avoid standing or sitting for long periods and to distrib-ute body weight by altering stance.

     g.    Leg cramps: Increase calcium and decrease phosphorus intake, evaluate diet, and apply heat to muscles; also dor-siflex foot and press knee downward.

     h.    Faintness: Instruct client to move slowly, avoid crowds, and remain in a cool environment.

     i.    Shortness of breath: Encourage proper posture and use of pillows behind head and shoulders at night; instruct client on rib cage lightening to increase flexibility of in-tercostal muscles.

     j.    Difficulty sleeping: Encourage a warm, caffeine-free drink before bed and relaxation techniques.

**3.**    Help the couple deal with sexual changes and concerns.

**4.**    Review the plan for labor and delivery:
     a.    Plan for analgesia or anesthesia
     b.    Breathing and relaxation methods
     c.    Monitoring equipment
     d.    Tour of labor and delivery area
     e.    Plans for feeding

**G.**  **Evaluation**

  **1.**    Maternal weight gain and nutritional status are within normal limits.

  **2.**    Client reports increased comfort and understanding of preg-nancy.

  **3.**    Client reports adequate elimination patterns.

  **4.**    Fetal growth is within normal limits.

  **5.**    The client exhibits no signs of complications.

  **6.**    The client demonstrates positive adjustment to pregnancy.

  **7.**    The client or couple exhibits adequate preparation for labor and delivery.

# Bibliography

Bobak, I. M., & Jensen, M. D. (1993). *Maternity and gynecologic care: The nurse and the family* (5th ed.). St. Louis: C.V. Mosby.

Gorrie, T. M., McKinney, E. S., & Murray, S. S. (1994). *Foundations of maternal newborn nursing.* Philadelphia: W.B. Saunders.

May, K. A., & Mahlmeister, L. R. (1994). *Maternal and neonatal nursing: Family-centered care* (3rd ed.). Philadelphia: J.B. Lippincott.

McElmurry, B. J., & Parker, R. S. (Ed.). (1993). *Annual review of women's health.* New York: National League for Nursing.

Olds, S. B., London, M. L., & Ladewig, P. W. (1992). *Maternal-newborn nursing: A family centered approach* (4th ed.). Menlo Park, CA: Addison-Wesley.

Reeder, S. J., Martin, L. L., & Koniak, D. (1992). *Maternity nursing: Family newborn, and women's health care* (17th ed.). Philadelphia: J.B. Lippincott.

# STUDY QUESTIONS

1. Which of the following is an expected outcome of antepartum care?
   a. To perform trimester-specific physiologic and psychosocial assessment
   b. To increase the expectant mother's and family's knowledge of pregnancy
   c. To provide education and counseling for the pregnant woman and her family
   d. To assess the client's experiences in relation to previous pregnancies and cultural expectations

2. Select from the following the nursing responsibility related to antepartum care:
   a. To assist all family members to experience pregnancy in a positive way
   b. To promote the successful integration of the newborn into the family
   c. To provide education and counseling for the pregnant woman and her family
   d. To increase the expectant mother's and father's knowledge of pregnancy

3. Which of the following would cause a false-positive result on a pregnancy test?
   a. The test was performed less than 10 days after an abortion.
   b. The test was performed too early or too late in the pregnancy.
   c. The urine sample was stored too long at room temperature.
   d. A spontaneous abortion (or a missed abortion) is impending.

4. FHR can be auscultated with a fetoscope as early as
   a. 5 weeks' gestation
   b. 10 weeks' gestation
   c. 15 weeks' gestation
   d. 20 weeks' gestation

5. Ultrasonography provides different information during each trimester. For which of the following purposes would it be typically used in the third trimester?
   a. To evaluate the fetus for possible congenital anomalies
   b. To determine the fetal position and obtain an estimate of size
   c. To confirm suspected multiple gestation
   d. To enhance prenatal testing and evaluation of pelvic mass

6. Quickening in primagravidas usually can be detected during which of the following weeks of gestation?
   a. 15 to 17 weeks
   b. 10 to 14 weeks
   c. 18 to 20 weeks
   d. 20 to 22 weeks

7. EFHM is performed during the NST or the CST. Which of the following best characterizes the CST?
   a. The fetus typically is monitored for at least 40 minutes; then the entire monitoring strip (or tracing) is analyzed.
   b. Any abnormal or nonreactive stress test results require further evaluation that same day.
   c. It is the least invasive test of fetal well-being that involves using an electronic fetal monitor.
   d. Three contractions within 10 minutes must be evaluated. Ideally, each contraction should last from 40 to 60 seconds.

8. A client's LMP began August 28. Her EDD should be which of the following?
   a. May 10
   b. April 28
   c. May 21
   d. June 4

9. Uterine size is reported in terms of weeks of gestation when the LMP is unknown. Which of the following fundal heights indicates less than 12 weeks' gestation?
   a. Presence of the uterus in the pelvis
   b. Presence of the uterus on sonogram
   c. Presence of the uterus in the abdomen

d. Presence of the uterus at the umbilicus

10. Which group of danger signals should be reported promptly during the antepartum period?
    a. Constipation, nausea, cramping, rapid weight gain
    b. Breast enlargement, headache, cramping, and urinary frequency
    c. Spotting, blurred vision, nasal stuffiness, breast tenderness
    d. Vaginal bleeding, blurred vision, and leaking of amniotic fluid

For additional questions, see
*Lippincott's Self-Study Series* Software
Available at your bookstore

# ANSWER KEY

**1. Correct response: b**
One of the expected outcomes of antepartum care is increased parental knowledge about pregnancy.
**a and c.** These are nursing responsibilities.
**d.** This is a factor affecting the antepartum experience.
*Knowledge/Health Promotion/*
*Evaluation*

**2. Correct response: c**
One of the nursing responsibilities during antepartum care is to provide education and counseling for the pregnant woman and her family.
**a, b, and d.** These are all goals or factors affecting the antepartum experience.
*Application/Safe Care/Implementation*

**3. Correct response: a**
A false-positive reaction can occur if the pregnancy test is performed less than 10 days after an abortion.
**b, c, and d.** These can all produce false-negative results.
*Knowledge/Physiologic/Implementation*

**4. Correct response: d**
The FHR can be auscultated with a fetoscope at about 20 weeks' gestation.
**a, b, and c.** Are all incorrect answers.
*Knowledge/Physiologic/Assessment (Dx)*

**5. Correct response: b**
Ultrasonography may be used in the third trimester to determine the size of the fetus and its position.
**a, c, and d.** These are typical uses of ultrasonography in the first and second trimesters.
*Knowledge/Physiologic/Assessment*

**6. Correct response: c**
Quickening in primagravidas can usually be detected between 18 and 20 weeks' gestation.

**a, b, and d.** Are all incorrect for primagravidas, although fetal movement can be detected as early as 16 weeks in multigravidas.
*Knowledge/Physiologic/Assessment (Dx)*

**7. Correct response: d**
During the CST, three contractions within 10 minutes—ideally, each lasting 40 to 60 seconds—must be evaluated to assess fetal response to stress.
**a, b, and c.** These are characteristics of NST.
*Knowledge/Physiologic/Implementation*

**8. Correct response: c**
Dating pregnancy when LMP is known by Nägele's rule: to the first day of the LMP, add 7 days, subtract 3 months, and add 1 year (if applicable) to arrive at the EDD.
**a, b, and d.** Are all incorrect dates.
*Physiologic/Application/Assessment (Dx)*

**9. Correct response: a**
When the LMP is unknown, the gestational age of the fetus is estimated by uterine size or position (fundal height). Presence of the uterus in the pelvis indicates less than 12 weeks' gestation.
**b, c, and d.** All are incorrect.
*Application/Physiologic/Assessment*

**10. Correct response: d**
The group of danger signals that should be reported include, vaginal bleeding, blurred vision, leaking of amniotic fluid, rapid weight gain, and elevated blood pressure.
**a, b, and c.** All are incorrect. These groups of signs and symptoms may all occur at one time or another but are more characteristic of discomfort than danger.
*Analysis/Health Promotion/*
*Implementation*

# *Intrapartum Care*

## I. Overview

### A. Intrapartum care

1. The intrapartum period extends from the beginning of contractions that cause cervical dilation to the first 1 to 4 hours after delivery of the newborn and placenta.

117

2. Intrapartum care refers to the medical and nursing care given to a pregnant client and family during labor and delivery.

**B. Goals of intrapartum care**

1. To promote greatest physical and emotional well-being in the mother and fetus
2. To incorporate family-centered care concepts into the labor and delivery experience

**C. Factors affecting the intrapartum experience**

1. Previous experience with pregnancy
2. Cultural and personal expectations
3. Prepregnant health and biophysical preparedness for childbearing
4. Motivation for childbearing
5. Socioeconomic readiness
6. Age of mother, partnered versus unpartnered status, accessibility of prenatal care
7. Extent of childbirth education

**D. Nursing responsibilities**

1. Determine maternal and fetal well-being on admission to the labor and delivery setting.
2. Establish a welcoming environment that demonstrates to the client and family that quality care will be provided.
3. Provide appropriate, clear, concise explanations about the physical surroundings, procedures, and expectations.

 4. **Make timely, accurate assessments, and perform interventions appropriate to the labor and delivery experience. Carefully document all nursing care and information.**

**II. Phenomena and processes of labor and delivery**

**A. Onset of labor**

1. **Labor is the process by which the fetus and products of conception are expelled as the result of regular, progressive, frequent, and strong uterine contractions.**
2. Theoretically, labor is thought to result from:
   a. Progesterone deprivation
   b. Oxytocin stimulation
   c. Fetal endocrine control
   d. Uterine decidua activation (a complex cascade of bioactive chemical agents into the amniotic fluid)

**B. Factors affecting labor**

1. *Passageway* refers to the pelvis and birth canal; factors include:
   a. Type of pelvis (eg, gynecoid, android, anthropoid, platypelloid)

  b. Structure of pelvis (eg, true versus false pelvis)
  c. Pelvic inlet diameters
  d. Pelvic outlet diameters
  e. Ability of the uterine segment to distend, the cervix to dilate, and the vaginal canal and introitus to distend

2. *Passenger* refers to the fetus and its ability to move through the passageway; this is based on:
   a. Size of the fetal head and capability of the head to mold to the passageway
   b. Fetal presentation—the part of the fetus that enters the maternal pelvis first (eg, cephalic [vertex, face, brow], breech [frank, single or double footling, complete], shoulder [transverse lie])
   c. Fetal attitude—the relationship of fetal parts to one another

   d. **Fetal position—the relationship of a particular reference point of the presenting part and the maternal pelvis, described with a series of three letters (ie, side of maternal pelvis [L, left; R, right; T, transverse], presenting part [O, occiput; S, sacrum; Sc, scapula; M, mentum], and part of the maternal pelvis [A, anterior; P, posterior]; Fig. 9-1).**

3. *Power* refers to the frequency, duration, and strength of uterine contractions to cause complete cervical effacement and dilation.
4. *Placental factors* refer to the site of placental insertion.
5. *Psyche* refers to the client's psychological state, available support systems, preparation for childbirth, experiences, and coping strategies.

C. **Signs and symptoms of impending labor (premonitory signs)**
  1. Lightening: descent of the fetus and uterus into the pelvic cavity 2 to 3 weeks before onset of labor
  2. Braxton Hicks contractions: irregular, intermittent contractions that have occurred during pregnancy, become uncomfortable, and produce a drawing pain in the abdomen and groin
  3. Cervical changes: softening, "ripening," and effacement of the cervix that will cause expulsion of the mucus plug (bloody show)

  4. **Rupture of membranes: amniotic membranes that may rupture before the onset of labor (If the woman suspects that her membranes have ruptured, she should contact her health care provider and go to the labor suite imme-**

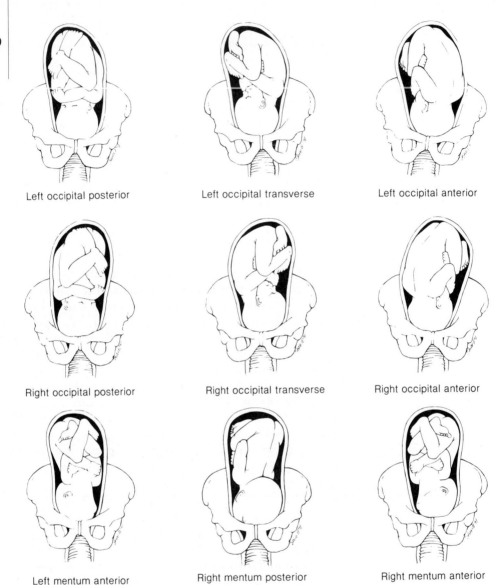

Left occipital posterior      Left occipital transverse      Left occipital anterior

Right occipital posterior      Right occipital transverse      Right occipital anterior

Left mentum anterior      Right mentum posterior      Right mentum anterior

**FIGURE 9–1.**
Fetal positions.

diately so that she may be examined for prolapsed cord—
a life-threatening condition for the fetus.)

5. Burst of energy or increased tension and fatigue
6. Weight loss of about 1 to 3 lb 2 to 3 days before onset of labor

**D.** **Characteristics of true labor**
1. Contractions occur at regular intervals.
2. Contractions start in the back and sweep around to the abdomen, increase in intensity and duration, and gradually have shortened intervals.
3. Contractions are intensified by walking.
4. "Bloody show" is usually present (pink-tinged mucus released from the cervical canal as labor starts).

5. **Cervix becomes effaced and dilated.**
6. Sedation does not stop contractions.

**E.** **Characteristics of false labor**
1. Contractions occur at irregular intervals.
2. Located chiefly in abdomen, the intensity remains the same or is variable; intervals remain long.
3. Walking has no intensifying effect and often gives relief.
4. Bloody show usually is not present. If present, it is usually brownish rather than bright red and may be due to recent pelvic examination or intercourse.

5. **Cervix evidences no change.**
6. Sedation tends to decrease number of contractions.

**F.** **Stages of labor**
1. First stage of labor

   a. **Begins with the onset of regular contractions, which cause progressive cervical dilation and effacement; ends when the cervix is completely effaced and dilated.**
   b. Latent phase: begins with onset of regular contractions and effacement and dilation of the cervix to 3 to 4 cm; it lasts an average of 6.4 hours for nulliparas and 4.8 hours for multiparas; contractions become increasingly stronger and more frequent.
   c. Active phase: dilation continues from 3 to 4 cm to complete dilation (10 cm); contractions become stronger, more frequent, longer, and more painful. This active period has three phases:

   ► Acceleration phase
   ► Phase of maximum slope
   ► Declaration or transition phase

   d. The interval between 8 and 10 cm dilation also is referred to as the transition phase.
   e. The culmination of the active phase is the deceleration phase (9–10 cm), when the woman feels more relaxed

and perceives less discomfort, or the intensity, frequency, and duration of contractions may peak with an irresistible urge to push.

**2.** Second stage (expulsive stage)

    a. **Stage begins with complete dilation of cervix and ends with delivery of newborn; duration may differ among primiparas (longer) and multiparas (shorter).**

    b. Contractions are severe at 2- to 3-minute intervals, with a duration of 50 to 90 seconds.

    c. This stage should be completed within 1 hour after complete dilation.

    d. Newborn exits birth canal by cardinal movements or mechanisms of labor (Fig. 9-2):

       ▶ Descent
       ▶ Flexion
       ▶ Internal rotation
       ▶ Extension
       ▶ Restitution
       ▶ External rotation
       ▶ Expulsion

    e. **"Crowning" occurs when newborn's head or presenting part appears at the vaginal opening.**

    f. Episiotomy (surgical incision in perineum) may be done to facilitate delivery and avoid laceration of perineum.

**3.** Third stage (placental stage)

    a. **This stage begins with delivery of newborn and ends with delivery of placenta.**

    b. Stage occurs in two phases: placental separation and placental expulsion.

    c. Signs of placental separation include uterus becoming globular, fundus rising in abdomen, cord lengthening, and increasing bleeding (trickle or gush).

    d. Contraction of the uterus controls uterine bleeding and aids with placental separation and expulsion.

    e. Generally, oxytocic drugs are administered to help contract uterus.

**4. Fourth stage (recovery and bonding)**

    a. Stage lasts 1 to 4 hours after birth.

    b. Mother and newborn recover from the physical process of birth.

    c. Maternal organs undergo initial readjustment to the nonpregnant state.

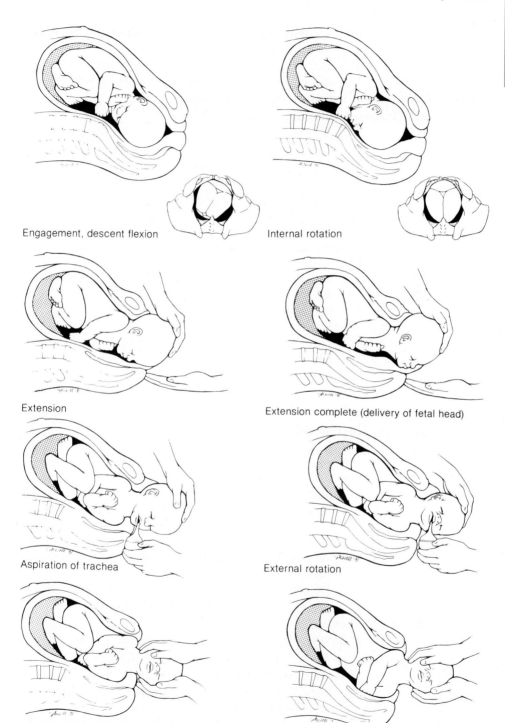

Engagement, descent flexion

Internal rotation

Extension

Extension complete (delivery of fetal head)

Aspiration of trachea

External rotation

Delivery of shoulders

Expulsion

**FIGURE 9–2.**
Cardinal movements of labor.

      d.    Newborn body systems begin to adjust to extrauterine life and stabilize.

      e.    Uterus contracts in midline of abdomen with fundus midway between umbilicus and symphysis pubis.

## III. Essentials of intrapartum assessment

### A. Maternal status and progress of labor

1. History: name, age, physician, weight, allergies, blood type and Rh, previous medical conditions, prenatal problems, gravida and para status, estimated date of delivery (EDD), prenatal education, and method of newborn feeding
2. Risk factor screens: bleeding, premature rupture of membranes, hydramnios, abnormal presentation, multiple gestation, prolapsed cord, precipitous labor, meconium-stained amniotic fluid, fetal heart irregularities, postmaturity
3. Physiologic assessment:
   a. Maternal vital signs, weight, cardiac and respiratory status
   b. Fundal height
   c. Status of labor: contractions (onset, frequency, duration, intensity), membranes, bleeding, cervical dilation, fetal descent
   d. Laboratory findings
4. Psychosocial status (eg, anxiety, childbirth education, support systems, response to labor)
5. **Assessment of labor progress:**
   a. **Palpation or electronic monitoring (external with tocodynamometer and internal with intrauterine pressure catheter) to assess the duration, frequency, and intensity of contractions**
   b. **Vaginal examination to assess cervical dilation (opening of external os from closed to 10 mm) and cervical effacement (thinning and shortening of the cervix), as measured from 0% (thick) to 100% (paper thin) effaced**
   c. **Determination of station—the relationship of the presenting part to the pelvic ischial spines**

### B. Fetal assessment

1. Inspect the maternal abdomen to determine fetal lie—the relationship of the long axis (spine) of the fetus to the long axis of the mother. Lies include:
   a. Longitudinal lie: Long axis of fetus is parallel to the long axis of the mother.
   b. Transverse lie: Long axis of fetus is perpendicular to the long axis of the mother.

2. Palpate the abdomen using the four Leopold maneuvers to determine fetal position and its possible size.
3. Monitor fetal status.
   a. Auscultate fetal heart rate (FHR):

   ▶ **Normal range: 120 to 160 beats/min**
   ▶ Decreases during contractions but returns to normal after 10 to 15 seconds

   b. Assess changes in FHR to identify:

   ▶ **Early deceleration: slowing of FHR early in contraction; considered benign; mirrors contraction; indication of head compression**

   ▶ **Late deceleration: indication of fetal hypoxia; usually begins at acme and ends after contraction; indicates utero-placental insufficiency**

   ▶ **Variable deceleration: transient decrease in FHR before, during, or after contraction; indicates cord compression; characteristic "V" or "U" pattern**
   ▶ Bradycardia: FHR < 100 beats/min or a drop of 20 beats/min below baseline; indicates cord compression or placental separation
   ▶ Tachycardia: FHR > 160 beats/min; indicates fetal distress if persistent for more than 1 hour or accompanied by late deceleration
   ▶ Loss of beat-to-beat variability: indicates fetal reaction to maternal drugs, fetal sleep, or fetal demise

   c. Assess fetal acid–base status with fetal blood sampling or fetal scalp stimulation

## IV. Intrapartum pain management
### A. Overview of pain
1. Intrapartum pain is a subjective experience of physical sensations associated with uterine contractions, cervical dilation and effacement, and fetal descent during labor and birth.
2. Physiologic responses to pain may include increased blood pressure, pulse, respirations, perspiration, pupil diameter, muscle tension (facial tension, fisted hands) or muscle activity (eg, pacing, turning, twisting).
3. Nonverbal expressions of pain may include withdrawal, hostility, fear, depression.
4. Verbal expression may include statements of pain, moaning, and groaning.
5. Pain relief may be achieved by using prepared childbirth methods (eg, Lamaze), analgesics, or regional anesthetics
6. Intervention for pain relief during labor depends on such factors as:

        a. Gestational age of fetus

        b. Frequency, duration, and intensity of contractions

        c. Labor progress

        d. Maternal response to pain and labor

        e. Allergies and sensitivities to analgesics and anesthetics

**B. Goals of pain management**

1. To provide maximal relief of pain with maximal safety for mother and fetus
2. To facilitate labor and delivery as a positive family experience

**C. Factors affecting perception of intrapartum pain**

1. Previous experience with painful stimuli and personal expectations for the birth experience
2. Cultural concept of pain, specifically during childbirth, and how one should respond
3. Rapidly progressive uterine contractions
4. Fear, anxiety, fatigue

**D. Causes of intrapartum pain**

1. Uterine anoxia due to compressed muscle cells during contraction
2. Compression of the nerve ganglia in the cervix and lower uterine segment during contraction
3. Stretching of cervix during dilation and effacement
4. Traction on, stretching, and displacement of the perineum
5. Pressure on urethra, bladder, rectum during fetal descent
6. Distention of the lower uterine segment
7. Stretching of the uterine ligaments

**E. Nursing responsibilities**

1. Collaborate with client and birth attendant to determine the most effective method of pain relief during each stage and phase of the intrapartum period

**𝓶 2. Continually assess the client's response to labor and the need for comfort, analgesia, or anesthesia**

**𝓶 3. Continually assess fetal response to labor and pain relief methods used**

**F. Nonpharmacologic pain relief**

1. Prepared childbirth methods can help the client feel more in control and relaxed, helping her "work with" the contractions; it may shorten labor.
2. Hypnosis may be useful in some clients.
3. Interventions aimed at supporting the client during labor may be helpful, such as:

        a. Providing information about the progress of labor

        b.   Reinforcing techniques learned in prepared childbirth classes

        c.   Directing breathing methods, abdominal lifting, pushing, relieving external pressure, distraction, cutaneous stimulation, and relaxation

**G.** **Pharmacologic pain relief**

  1.   Analgesia

        a.   Obstetric analgesia may include the use of narcotic analgesics (eg, morphine, meperidine), sedative-hypnotics (eg, barbiturates), or tranquilizers.

        b.   Narcotic analgesics provide effective pain relief and slight sedation.

        c.   **Narcotic analgesics are systemic drugs that readily cross the placental barrier, with depressive effects on the neonate occurring 2 to 3 hours after intramuscular injection.**

        d.   Maternal side effects include nausea, vomiting, mild respiratory depression, and transient mental impairment.

        e.   Narcotic antagonists (ie, naloxone [Narcan]) must be readily available in case of respiratory depression in mother or newborn.

        f.   The decision to administer a narcotic analgesic is predicated on the results of a vaginal examination; if birth is anticipated within 2 to 3 hours, the risk of neonatal narcosis may preclude the use of analgesics.

        g.   Dosage is kept to the smallest effective dose.

  2.   Barbiturates

        a.   These drugs cause maternal sedation and relaxation.

        b.   Maternal side effects of barbiturates include nausea, vomiting, hypotension, restlessness, and vertigo.

        c.   **The rapid transfer of barbiturates across the placental barrier and lack of an antagonist makes them generally inappropriate during active labor.**

        d.   Neonatal side effects of barbiturates include central nervous system depression, prolonged drowsiness, delayed establishment of feeding (eg, due to poor sucking reflex or poor sucking pressure)

  3.   Tranquilizers

        a.   These drugs decrease the anxiety and apprehension associated with pain and sometimes relieve the nausea associated with narcotic analgesics.

        b.   Tranquilizers potentiate active sedative and analgesic effects, decreasing the dosage needed to produce the desired effect.

  c. Maternal side effects of tranquilizers include hypotension (which in turn decreases fetoplacental circulation), drowsiness, and dizziness.

  d. **Fetal effects of tranquilizers include tachycardia and loss of normal beat-to-beat variability on electronic fetal heart monitoring.**

  e. Newborn effects of tranquilizers include hypotonia, hypothermia, generalized drowsiness, and reluctance to feed for the first few days.

 **4.** Regional anesthesia (conduction anesthesia)

  a. Types include spinal block, epidural, paracervical, pudendal block, and local infiltration.

  b. These blocks provide pain relief with injected anesthetic agents at sensory nerve pathways.

  c. **Adverse reactions may include maternal hypotension, allergic or toxic reaction, respiratory paralysis, and partial or total anesthetic failure.**

  d. Nursing responsibilities during administration of regional anesthesia include assisting the anesthesiologist as requested, establishing a reliable intravenous line, and being prepared with medications and equipment for emergency situations if they arise.

 **5.** Systemic analgesics (eg, narcotics, tranquilizers, sedatives) must be timed carefully to minimize effects on the fetus.

 **6.** Inhalation anesthesia (eg, nitrous oxide, halothane) are used rarely.

 **7.** Rarely, general anesthesia (inhalant and intravenous) may be used in labor and delivery.

## V. Nursing management during first stage of labor

 **A.** Assessment

  **1.** Perform an initial assessment of labor status, covering:

   a. Gravida and para status

   b. EDD or estimated date of confinement

   c. Time of labor onset

   d. Frequency and duration of contractions

   e. Rupture of membranes, bloody show, or other signs of labor onset

  **2.** Document findings

  **3.** Assess maternal and fetal status, covering:

   a. FHR

   b. Status of amniotic membrane (If ruptured, determine time of rupture; note color and odor, if any.)

   c. Frequency, duration, and intensity of contractions

   d. Maternal vital signs

  e. Vaginal examination for cervical dilation and efface-ment, station, and position of fetal presenting part

  f. Maternal ability to cope with labor, available support people

**B.** **Nursing diagnoses**

  **1.** Ineffective Individual Coping

  **2.** Ineffective Family Coping: Compromised

  **3.** Fear

  **4.** Fluid Volume Deficit

  **5.** Knowledge Deficit

  **6.** Altered Nutrition: Less than body requirements

  **7.** Altered Oral Mucous Membrane

  **8.** Self Care Deficit

  **9.** Sleep Pattern Disturbance

  **10.** Altered Tissue Perfusion

  **11.** Risk for Injury

  **12.** Pain

**C.** **Planning and implementation**

  **1.** On admission to the labor and delivery unit:

    a. Collect urine specimen and other samples for laboratory testing as prescribed (eg, hemoglobin, hematocrit, sero-logic test for syphilis, and type and crossmatch, if indi-cated).

    b. Perform perineal preparation and enema, if indicated.

    c. Notify attending physician or midwife, and report sta-tus.

    d. Provide support.

    e. Obtain informed consent from client.

  **2.** During the first stage, latent phase:

    a. Provide information on emotional and physical support; provide pleasant, comfortable surroundings.

    b. Assess individual needs.

    c. **Assess maternal temperature every 4 hours; in cases of ruptured membranes, assess every 2 hours.**

    d. Assess blood pressure (BP), pulse and respiration every hour. (If BP is > 140/90 or pulse is > 100, notify at-tending physician.)

    e. Assess uterine contractions (frequency, duration, and in-tensity) every 30 minutes.

    f. Assess FHR every 30 minutes.

    g. Assess cervical dilation, effacement, station, and position of presenting part.

    h. Assess status of membranes; if ruptured, assess color and odor of amniotic fluid. If membranes are ruptured and head is not engaged, position mother to prevent cord prolapse.

**ℳ**    i.    **Interpret changes in the electronic fetal and maternal monitor strip, and take appropriate action.**

3. During the first stage, active phase:
   a. Provide safety, comfort, information, and emotional and physical support.
   b. Provide support during contractions: Coach breathing, give back rubs, and provide cool cloths.
   c. Assess contractions (frequency, duration, and intensity) every 15 to 30 minutes.
   d. Assess maternal blood pressure, pulse rate, and respirations (depth, rate) every hour.
   e. Assess FHR every 15 minutes.
   f. Assess cervical dilation, effacement, station, and position of presenting part as warranted.
   g. Provide pharmacologic support as prescribed.
   h. Assess hydration status.

**ℳ**    i.    **Offer client an opportunity to void every 1 to 2 hours.**
   j. Assess status of membranes; if ruptured, assess whether the presenting part is engaged. If not, check for prolapsed cord and perform appropriate nursing interventions.
   k. Interpret changes on the electronic fetal and maternal monitor strip, and take appropriate action.

4. During the first stage, transition phase:
   a. Provide information, comfort, and emotional and physical support.
   b. Assess contractions (frequency, duration, and intensity) every 15 minutes.
   c. Assess maternal blood pressure, pulse rate, and respirations every 30 minutes.
   d. Assess FHR every 15 minutes.
   e. Interpret changes on the electronic fetal and maternal monitor strip, and take appropriate action if indicated.
   f. Assess cervical dilation, effacement, station, and position of presenting part; with complete dilation, the fetus descends in the birth canal, and the client feels increased rectal pressure or the urge to push.

**D.** **Evaluation**
   1. The pregnant client experiences regular contractions and progresses to complete dilation.

2. The pregnant client can begin pushing when completely dilated to aid descent of the presenting fetal part.
3. The client's support system, nurses, and physician support her physically and emotionally to prepare for delivery.
4. The client works effectively with contractions to facilitate delivery.
5. Vital signs, FHR remain within normal limits.
6. Hydration and elimination are adequate.
7. Support person is physically and emotionally prepared.

## VI. Nursing management during second stage of labor

### A. Assessment

1. Evaluate contractions for frequency, duration, and intensity. (Normal parameters include strong contractions every 2–3 minutes, each lasting 45–90 seconds.)
2. Measure and record maternal blood pressure and pulse rate and FHR every 5 to 15 minutes.
3. Perform sterile vaginal examination to determine progress.
4. Interpret electronic fetal and maternal monitoring strip for changes.

### B. Nursing diagnoses

1. Risk for Ineffective Airway Clearance (newborn)
2. Ineffective Individual or Family Coping (mother, other family members)
3. Fear (mother)
4. Fluid Volume Deficit (mother)
5. Hypoxia (newborn)
6. Knowledge Deficit (mother or family)
7. Altered Oral Mucous Membrane (mother)
8. Pain (mother)
9. Self Care Deficit (mother)
10. Altered Tissue Perfusion (mother)

### C. Planning and implementation

1. Notify physician or nurse-midwife; provide emotional and physical support and comfort measures, and explain labor process and progress.
2. Assist the client with pushing as indicated.
3. Prepare delivery area with equipment and supplies.
4. Prepare for delivery when perineal area is bulging in a primipara and when the cervix is dilated 7 to 8 cm in a multipara.
5. Place the client in the birthing position.
6. Assist attending physician or nurse midwife with birth; help support person to be supportive, and check all vital signs and FHR.
7. Establish and maintain a patent airway; suction with a bulb

syringe or a DeLee mucus trap, and place the newborn on his or her side.

8. Compensate for poor newborn thermoregulation:
   a. Dry immediately with warm blanket.
   b. Place under radiant warmer.
   c. Wrap in warmed dry blanket or place on mother's skin.

9. **Determine Apgar score at 1 and 5 minutes after delivery (Fig. 9-3).**

10. Inspect the umbilical cord for two arteries and one vein.

11. Weigh and measure the newborn as his or her condition stabilizes.

12. Footprint the newborn, and fingerprint the mother.

13. Record the newborn's first voiding and stool passage.

14. Assess the newborn's gestational age.

15. Administer prophylactic eye medication to protect the conjunctivae from infection.

16. Administer vitamin K (phytonadione [Aquamephyton]) if prescribed.

**D. Evaluation**

1. The client verbalizes understanding of the interventions used to promote comfort.

**APGAR SCORING CHART**

| SIGN | SCORE 0 | SCORE 1 | SCORE 2 |
|---|---|---|---|
| Heart rate | Absent | Slow (<100) | >100 |
| Respiratory effort | Absent | Slow, irregular; weak cry | Good; strong cry |
| Muscle tone | Flaccid | Some flexion of extremities | Well flexed |
| Reflex irritability | | | |
|   Response to catheter in nostril | No reponse | Grimace | Cough or sneeze |
|     or | | | |
|   Slap to sole of foot | No response | Grimace | Cry and withdrawal of foot |
| Color | Blue, pale | Body pink, extremities blue | Completely pink |

*(From Apgar V., et al. (1958). Evaluation of the newborn infant: Second report. Journal of the American Medical Association, 168, 1985. Copyright 1958, American Medical Association; with permission.)*

**FIGURE 9–3.**
The nurse and other members of the healthcare team use the Apgar score to measure the newborn's immediate adjustment to extrauterine life. Scores are assigned at 1 minute and again at 5 minutes after birth. Each sign is assigned a value. A score from 7 to 10 indicates that the newborn is doing well. A score of 4 or less indicates that the newborn may need assistance.

2. The client verbalizes a decrease in discomfort and shows signs of relaxing between explusive efforts.
3. The client and support person verbalize a decrease in anxiety.
4. The client uses effective breathing and expulsive techniques.
5. The client assumes a position that facilitates expulsive efforts, maintains placental perfusion, and prevents or alleviates cord compression.
6. The newborn breathes spontaneously with a minimum of respiratory effort.
7. The newborn maintains skin temperature between 36.4°C and 37.2°C (97.5°–99°F) in the first hour after delivery.

## VII. Nursing management during third stage of labor
### A. Assessment
1. Evaluate maternal physiologic adjustment:
   a. Vital signs
   b. Uterine firmness
   c. Amount, color of lochia
2. Assess the new mother's emotional adjustment.

### B. Nursing diagnoses
1. Knowledge Deficit
2. Altered Oral Mucous Membrane
3. Pain
4. Self Care Deficit

### C. Planning and implementation
1. Promote physiologic adaptation by the new mother.
2. Initiate fundal massage gently with adequate support to the lower uterine segment.

3. **Promote parent–newborn interaction by placing the newborn on the mother's abdomen and encouraging parents to touch the newborn.**
4. Monitor mother and newborn for potential complications.
5. Document intrapartum care, for example:
   a. Time of delivery of newborn and placenta
   b. 1- and 5-minute Apgar scores
   c. Any immediate neonatal care provided
   d. Extent and repair of perineal lacerations or episiotomy
   e. Estimated maternal blood loss
   f. Medications administered before, during, and after delivery (to mother and neonate)
   g. Placement of identification bands, footprinting and fingerprinting
   h. Maternal and newborn vital signs

### D. Evaluation

1. Maternal bleeding is within normal limits with firm uterine tone and normal maternal vital signs.
2. The new mother verbalizes comfort with fundal massage.
3. Parents and newborn begin interaction by face-to-face gazing and parental exploration of newborn.

 4. **Complications, if any, are promptly identified, and appropriate actions are taken.**
5. Documentation of intrapartum care is accurate and complete.

**VIII.** **Nursing management during fourth stage of labor**

**A.** **Assessment**

1. Assess the mother's vital signs, bladder, fundus, perineum, and lochia.
2. Observe newborn for respiratory effort and maintenance of body temperature.
3. Observe for signs of parent–newborn attachment.
4. Evaluate mother's and newborn's breast-feeding attempts if mother is breast-feeding.

**B.** **Nursing Diagnoses**

1. Knowledge Deficit
2. Self Care Deficit
3. Anxiety
4. Ineffective Coping
5. Powerlessness
6. Risk for Injury
7. Pain

**C.** **Planning and Implementation**

1. Provide comfort measures for afterpains or perineal discomfort (eg, analgesics, ice packs, opportunity to void).
2. Place a warm blanket over the mother and newborn.
3. Offer mother warm liquids of her choice.
4. Suction secretions from the newborn's nose and mouth as necessary to maintain respirations.
5. Maintain newborn's temperature by placing in skin-to-skin contact with mother, covering with warm blankets, or using a radiant warmer.
6. Assist mother to breast-feed her newborn if she is breast-feeding.
7. Promote family integration when parents are ready by inviting siblings and other family members into the room.
8. Help younger siblings to see and hold the newborn when possible. (Toddlers are usually more interested in their mother than in the newborn.)
9. Continue to observe mother and newborn for potential complications.

    **10.** Document intrapartum care:
       a.  Neonatal care given
       b.  Maternal condition related to discomfort, bleeding, vital signs
       c.  Maternal or newborn elimination—voiding or bowel elimination
       d.  Medications administered to mother or newborn
       e.  Newborn's vital signs
       f.  Maternal and newborn breast-feeding attempts and responses
       g.  Newborn condition when transferred to nursery
       h.  Maternal condition when transferred to postpartum unit

**D.** **Evaluation**
    **1.** The newborn maintains normal respirations and body temperature.
    **2.** See Section VII, D.

## Bibliography

Bobak, I. M., & Jensen, M. D. (1993). *Maternity and gynecologic care: The nurse and the family* (5th ed.). St. Louis: C.V. Mosby.

May, K. A., & Mahlmeister, L. R. (1994). *Maternal and neonatal nursing: Family-centered care* (3rd ed.). Philadelphia: J.B. Lippincott.

McElmurry, B. J., & Parker, R. S. (Ed.) (1993). *Annual review of women's health.* New York: National League for Nursing.

Olds, S. B., London, M. L., & Ladewig, P. W. (1992). *Maternal-newborn nursing: A family centered approach* (4th ed.). Menlo Park, CA: Addison-Wesley.

Reeder, S. J., Martin, L. L., & Koniak, D. (1992). *Maternity nursing: Family newborn, and women's health care* (17th ed.). Philadelphia: J.B. Lippincott.

## STUDY QUESTIONS

1. From the following, select the best definition of intrapartum care:
   a. It tries to promote the greatest physical and emotional well-being in the mother and fetus.
   b. It incorporates family-centered care concepts into the labor and delivery experience.
   c. It extends from the beginning of contractions to the first 1 to 4 hours after delivery of the newborn and placenta.
   d. It extends from the beginning of the pregnancy through the delivery of the newborn and the first 1 to 4 days after the delivery.

2. Which of the following is a nursing responsibility during intrapartum care?
   a. To assess maternal and fetal well-being on admission to the labor and delivery setting
   b. To discuss maternal and fetal well-being on admission to the labor and delivery setting
   c. To define the mother's previous experiences during labor and admission and delivery periods
   d. To determine the mother's and partner's preparedness to care for the newborn after delivery

3. Several factors affect labor. Which of the following factors refers to the passageway?
   a. Size of the fetal head and its ability to mold to the maternal pelvis
   b. The presentation of the fetus in relation to the maternal pelvis
   c. The structure of the maternal pelvis (eg, gynecoid versus android)
   d. The fetal attitude and the relationship of fetal parts to one another

4. There are many essential intrapartum assessments. Which of the following relates to fetal assessment?
   a. Assess the phases, duration, frequency, and intensity of the contractions to determine the stage of delivery.
   b. Inspect the maternal abdomen to determine fetal lie—the relationship of the spine of the fetus to the long axis of the mother.
   c. Perform a vaginal examination to assess cervical dilation and effacement and to determine the station of the fetus.
   d. Perform a psychosocial assessment of the mother to determine her knowledge related to childbirth education.

5. The fetal position is described by a series of letters. The first letter in the series denotes which of the following?
   a. The presenting part of the fetus
   b. The side of the maternal pelvis
   c. The size of the maternal pelvis
   d. The type of delivery of the fetus

6. Which of the following are characteristics of true labor?
   a. Contractions are irregular, and the intensity remains the same.
   b. Contractions are regular, and the intensity remains the same.
   c. Contractions occur at regular intervals and are not intensified by walking.
   d. Contractions occur at regular intervals and are intensified by walking.

7. During which stage of labor does "crowning" occur?
   a. First stage
   b. Second stage
   c. Third stage
   d. Fourth stage

8. Which of the following is a goal of pain management during labor and delivery?
   a. To assess continually maternal response to labor and the need for comfort, analgesia, or anesthesia
   b. To assess continually fetal response to labor and methods used to relieve maternal pain
   c. To assess previous maternal experi-

ence with painful stimuli and personal expectations for the childbirth experience

d. To provide maximal relief of pain with maximal safety for the mother and fetus and to facilitate labor and delivery

9. Barbiturates are usually not given for pain relief during labor because:
   a. the neonatal effects include hypotonia, hypothermia, generalized drowsiness, and reluctance to feed for the first few days.
   b. these drugs readily cross the placental barrier, causing depressive effects in the newborn 2 to 3 hours after intramuscular injection.
   c. they rapidly transfer across the placenta, and lack of an antagonist make them generally inappropriate during labor.
   d. Adverse reactions may include maternal hypotension, allergic or toxic reaction, or partial or total respiratory failure.

10. Nursing management during all stages of labor includes assessment. Which of the following occurs during the third stage of labor?
    a. Evaluation of maternal physiologic adjustment, covering such factors as vital signs, uterine firmness, and the amount and color of lochia
    b. Determination of the mother's gravida and para status, EDD, time of onset, frequency and duration of contractions, and bloody show
    c. Evaluation of contractions for frequency, duration, and intensity and monitoring of maternal blood pressure and pulse and FHR every 5 to 15 minutes
    d. Notification of the physician or midwife, provision of physical and emotional support and comfort measures, and explanation of labor process and progress

For additional questions, see
*Lippincott's Self-Study Series* Software
Available at your bookstore

# ANSWER KEY

1. **Correct response: c**
The intrapartum period extends from the beginning of contractions that cause cervical dilation to the first 1 to 4 hours after delivery of the newborn and placenta.
**a and b.** These are goals of intrapartum care.
**d.** This is an incorrect answer.
*Knowledge/Safe Care/NA*

2. **Correct response: a**
A nursing responsibility during intrapartum care is to determine maternal and fetal well-being on admission to the labor and delivery setting.
**b, c, and d.** These are basically factors that affect the intrapartum experience.
*Knowledge/Safe Care/Implementation*

3. **Correct response: c**
A factor of labor that affects the passageway is the structure of the pelvis (eg, gynecoid versus android).
**a, b, and d.** These relate to the fetus (passenger).
*Application/Physiologic/NA*

4. **Correct response: b**
One of the essential fetal assessments is inspection of the maternal abdomen to determine fetal lie—the relationship of the long axis (spine) of the fetus to the long axis of the mother.
**a, c, and d.** These are not fetal assessments.
*Application/Physiologic/Assessment*

5. **Correct response: b**
The first letter in the series relates to the side of the maternal pelvis (ie, L, left; R, right; or T, transverse).
**a, c, and d.** These are all incorrect answers.
*Comprehension/Physiologic/NA*

6. **Correct response: d**
In true labor, contractions occur at regular intervals and are intensified by walking.
**a, b, and c.** All are characteristics of false labor.
*Comprehension/Physiologic/NA*

7. **Correct response: b**
"Crowning" occurs during the second stage of labor.
**a, c, and d.** All are incorrect answers.
*Knowledge/Physiologic/NA*

8. **Correct response: d**
The goals of pain management are to provide maximal relief of pain with maximal safety for mother and fetus and to facilitate labor and delivery as a positive family experience.
**a, b, and c.** All are related to intrapartum pain but are not goals.
*Comprehension/Health Promotion/Evaluation*

9. **Correct response: c**
Pharmacologic pain relievers, such as barbiturates, rapidly cross the placental barrier. The lack of an antagonist for use in an emergency makes them generally inappropriate during labor.
**a, b, and d.** Refer to other types of medications.
*Application/Safe Care/Implementation*

10. **Correct response: a**
Nursing assessment during the third stage of labor includes the evaluation of maternal physiologic adjustment, covering such factors as vital signs, uterine firmness, and the color and amount of lochia.
**b, c, and d.** These assessments do not occur during the third stage of labor.
*Analysis/Physiologic/Assessment (Dx)*

# Postpartum Care

## I. Overview

### A. Essential concepts

1. Postpartum care refers to the medical and nursing care given to a client from the time of delivery until her body returns to its nonpregnant state.

2. **The puerperium is the 6-week period after delivery, beginning with termination of labor and ending with the return of the reproductive organs to the nonpregnant state.** It constitutes a physical and psychological adjustment to the process of childbearing.

3. Involution refers to the progressive changes in the uterus after delivery, leading to its return to near prepregnant size and condition.

4. This period is sometimes called the fourth trimester of pregnancy.
5. One aspect of postpartum care that commonly suffers with the trend toward earlier discharge is support in breast-feeding.

**B. Goals of postpartum care**
   1. Promote normal involution and return to the nonpregnant state.
   2. Prevent or minimize postpartum complications.
   3. Promote comfort and healing of pelvic, perianal, and perineal tissues.
   4. Assist in restoration of normal body functions.
   5. Increase understanding of physiologic and psychological changes.
   6. Facilitate newborn care and self-care by the new mother.
   7. Promote the newborn's successful integration into the family unit.
   8. Support parenting skills and parent–newborn attachment.

 9. **Provide effective discharge planning, including appropriate referral for home care follow-up.**

**C. Factors affecting the postpartum experience**
   1. Nature of labor and delivery and the birth outcome
   2. Preparation for labor and delivery and for parenting
   3. Abruptness of the transition to parenthood
   4. Family's individual and collective experiences with childbearing and childrearing
   5. Family members' role expectations
   6. Sensitivity and effectiveness of nursing and other professional care
   7. **Factors that increase the risk of postpartum complications include:**
      a. **Preeclampsia or eclampsia**
      b. **Diabetes**
      c. **Cardiac problems**
      d. **Uterine overdistention (eg, due to multiple births or hydramnios)**
      e. **Abruptio placentae or placenta previa**
      f. **Precipitous or prolonged labor, difficult delivery, extended time spent in stirrups**

**D. Nursing responsibilities**
   1. Provide sensitive professional care to the new parents:
      a. Accurate assessment of mother's physiologic and psychological status
      b. Anticipatory guidance and health teaching as needed
   2. Facilitate the family's bonding experience.

## II. Postpartum biophysical changes

### A. Reproductive system changes

1. The *uterus* contracts firmly, reducing its size by more than half; it remains this size for about 2 days, then decreases in size (involution) and descends about one finger breadth per day.

2. At 10 to 14 postpartum days, the uterus cannot be palpated abdominally. It returns to near its nonpregnant size by 4 to 6 postpartum weeks. The site of placental attachment requires 6 to 7 weeks to heal; endometrial regeneration requires 6 weeks.

3. **Lochia, discharge from the uterus during the first 3 weeks after delivery, occurs in three types:**

   a. *Lochia rubra:* dark red discharge occurring in the first 2 to 3 days, containing epithelial cells, erythrocytes, leukocytes, and decidua; has a characteristic odor

   b. *Lochia serosa:* pink to brownish discharge occurring from 3 to 10 days after delivery; serosanguineous discharge containing decidua, erythrocytes, leukocytes, cervical mucus, and microorganisms; has strong odor

   c. *Lochia alba:* almost colorless to creamy yellowish discharge, occurring from 10 days to 3 weeks after delivery and containing leukocytes, decidua, epithelial cells, fat, cervical mucus, cholesterol crystals, and bacteria; should have no odor

4. The *cervix* becomes thicker and firmer; by the end of the first postpartum week, it is still dilated about 1 cm. Complete cervical involution may take 3 to 4 months; childbirth results in a permanent change in the cervical os from round to elongated.

5. The *vagina* is smooth and swollen, with poor tone after delivery. Rugae reappear by 3 to 4 postpartum weeks, and the estrogen index returns in 6 to 10 weeks.

6. The *perineum* appears edematous and bruised after delivery; episiotomy or lacerations may be present.

7. The *abdomen* remains soft and flabby for some time after delivery. Striae remain but are silvery white. Diastasis recti (separation of abdominal recti muscles) may occur in women with poor muscle tone.

8. *Breast* changes include:

   a. Rapid drop in estrogen and progesterone levels with an increase in secretion of prolactin after delivery

   b. Colostrum at time of delivery; breast milk produced by the third or fourth postpartum day

   c. Larger and firmer breasts with lactation (primary engorgement), congestion subsiding in 1 or 2 days

9. In the breast, prolactin stimulates alveolar cells to produce milk. Sucking of newborn triggers release of oxytocin and con-

tractility of myoepithelial cells, which stimulate milk flow; this is known as the let-down reflex. The average amount of milk produced in 24 hours increases with time:

    a.   First week: 6 to 10 oz

    b.   1 to 4 weeks: 20 oz

    c.   After 4 weeks: 30 oz

**B.** **Endocrine system changes**

    **1.**   Estrogen and progesterone levels decrease rapidly after delivery.

    **2.**   Ovulation and resumption of menstruation are influenced by whether or not the client breast-feeds.

        a.   Lactating: 45% of women resume menstruation by 12 weeks; 80% have one or more anovulatory cycles before the first ovulation.

        b.   Nonlactating: 40% of women resume menstruation by 6 weeks after delivery, 65% by 12 weeks, and 90% by 24 weeks; 50% ovulate during the first cycle.

    **3.**   A rapid drop in estrogen and progesterone after delivery of the placenta is responsible for many of the anatomic and physiologic changes in the puerperium.

    **4.**   Requirements for rest and sleep increase significantly.

**C.** **Cardiovascular system changes**

    **1.**   Transient bradycardia (50–70 beats/min) occurs for 24 to 48 hours after delivery and may persist for the first 6 to 8 days.

    **2.**   Blood volume decreases to nonpregnant levels by 4 weeks after delivery.

    **3.**   Hematocrit rises by the third to seventh postpartum day.

    **4.**   Leukocytosis (20,000–30,000 white blood cells/mm$^3$) continues for several days after delivery.

    **5.**   Blood pressure remains stable; pulse returns to nonpregnant rate by 3 postpartum months.

**D.** **Immune system changes**

    **1.**   **Slight increases in maternal body temperature may occur without apparent cause following birth. However, the mother's temperature should remain within normal limits.**

    **2.**   **Any mother whose temperature reaches 38°C (100.4°F) in any two consecutive 24-hour periods during the first 10 postpartum days, excluding the first 24 postpartum hours, is considered to be febrile.**

**E.** **Respiratory system changes:** Pulmonary functions return to nonpregnant status by 6 months after delivery.

**F.** **Renal and urinary system changes**

    **1.**   Overdistention of the bladder is common due to increased bladder capacity, swelling, bruising of tissues around the urethra, and diminished sensation to increased pressure.

 **2. A full bladder will displace the uterus and can cause postpartum hemorrhage; bladder distention can lead to urinary retention.**

3. Adequate bladder emptying generally resumes in 5 to 7 days after tissue swelling and bruising resolve.

4. Glomerular filtration rate remains elevated for about 7 days after delivery.

5. Dilated ureters and renal pelvis return to their nonpregnant states in 6 to 10 weeks after delivery.

6. Puerperal diaphoresis and diuresis occur within the first 24 hours after delivery.

**G. Gastrointestinal system changes**

1. Hunger and thirst are common after delivery.

2. Gastrointestinal motility and tone return to the nonpregnant state within 2 weeks after delivery.

3. Constipation commonly occurs during the early postpartum period due to decreased intestinal muscle tone, perineal discomfort, and anxiety.

4. The client may return to her prepregnant weight in 6 to 8 weeks if weight gain during pregnancy was within the normal range.

5. Hemorrhoids are a common problem in the early postpartum period, due to pressure on the pelvic floor and straining during labor.

**H. Musculoskeletal system changes**

1. Most women ambulate 4 to 8 hours after delivery; early ambulation is encouraged to avoid complications, promote involution, and improve emotional outlook.

2. Relaxation and increased mobility of pelvic articulations occur 6 to 8 weeks after delivery.

**I. Integumentary system changes**

1. Melanin decreases gradually after delivery, causing decrease in hyperpigmentation. (Coloration may not return to prepregnant status, however.)

2. Visible vascular changes of pregnancy disappear as estrogen levels decrease.

## III. Postpartum psychosocial adaptation

**A. Essential concepts**

1. The postpartum period represents a time of emotional stress for the new mother, made even more difficult by the tremendous physiologic changes that occur.

2. Factors influencing successful transition to parenthood during the postpartum period include:
   a. Response and support of family and friends
   b. Relationship of the birthing experience to expectations and aspirations
   c. Previous childbearing and childrearing experiences
   d. Cultural influences

 3. **This period is described by Rubin as occurring in three stages: taking in, taking hold, and letting go.**

**B.** **Taking-in period**
1. During this period, occurring 1 to 2 days after delivery, the new mother typically is passive and dependent; energies are focused on bodily concerns.
2. She may review her labor and delivery experience frequently.
3. Uninterrupted sleep is important if the mother is to avoid the effects of sleep deprivation—fatigue, irritability, interference with normal restorative processes.
4. Additional nourishment may be needed, because the mother's appetite is usually increased; poor appetite may be a clue that the restorative process is not progressing normally.

**C.** **Taking-hold period**
1. During this period, extending from 2 to 4 days after delivery, the mother becomes concerned with her ability to parent successfully and accepts increasing responsibility for her newborn.
2. The mother focuses on regaining control over her body functions—bowel and bladder function, strength, and endurance.
3. The mother strives to master newborn care skills (eg, holding, breast-feeding or bottle feeding, bathing, diapering). She may be sensitive to feelings of inadequacy and may tend to perceive nurses' suggestions as overt or covert criticism. The nurse should take this into account when providing instruction and emotional support.

**D.** **Letting-go period**
1. This period generally occurs after the new mother returns home; it involves a time of family reorganization.
2. The mother assumes responsibility for newborn care; she must adapt to demands of the newborn's dependency and to her decreased autonomy, independence, and (typically) social interaction.
3. Postpartum depression most commonly occurs during this period.

**E.** **Postpartum depression**
1. Many mothers experience a "let down" feeling after giving birth, related to the magnitude of the birth experience and

doubts about the ability to cope effectively with the demands of childrearing.

2. **Typically, this depression is mild and transient, beginning 2 to 3 days after delivery and resolving within 1 to 2 weeks.**

3. Rarely, relatively mild depression leads to postpartum psychosis, a pathologic condition.

## IV. Nursing management during the normal postpartum period
### A. Assessment
1. Focus ongoing assessment on early identification of and prompt intervention for complications.
2. During the critical first hour after delivery, carefully assess for hemorrhage by checking the fundus frequently, inspecting the perineum for visible bleeding, and evaluating vital signs.
3. On subsequent postpartum assessments, include vital signs, fundus, lochia, perineum, breasts, elimination, nutrition, ambulation and exercise, rest and sleep patterns, and self-care and newborn care.
4. Assess temperature, blood pressure, pulse, and respirations every 4 to 8 hours during the first few days postpartum. Note especially:
   a. Mild temperature elevation, which may be due to dehydration, onset of lactation, or leukocytosis
   b. Hypotension with rapid, thready pulse (exceeding 100), which may signify hemorrhage and shock
   c. Orthostatic hypotension due to cardiovascular readjustment to the nonpregnant state
   d. Elevated blood pressure, possibly an early sign of pregnancy-induced hypertension
5. **Assess the fundus daily for firmness and location; make sure the client empties her bladder before palpating. Look for indications of subinvolution:**
   a. **Uterus not progressively decreasing in size or returning to the lower pelvis**
   b. **Uterus remaining flabby and poorly contracted**
   c. **Persistent backache or pelvic pain**
   d. **Heavy vaginal bleeding**
6. Assess the amount and character of lochia daily to provide an essential index of endometrial healing. Report any abnormal findings, such as:
   a. Fresh bleeding
   b. Heavy, persistent, and malodorous lochia rubra
7. Inspect the perineum, noting status of sutures (if any), tender-

ness, swelling, bruising, and hematoma; assess anal area for hemorrhoids and fissures.

8.  Assess breasts for firmness, tenderness, and warmth and nipples for cracks, fissures, and bleeding; handle breasts gently.
9.  Evaluate the client's level of knowledge about newborn feeding (breast-feeding and bottle feeding).
10. Assess degree of bladder distention often in the first 8 hours after delivery. Measure urine output; voiding small amounts on frequent, consecutive voidings indicates residual urine and possible need for catheterization.
11. Assess status of bowel elimination and the return to predelivery patterns.
12. Evaluate nutritional status, including ability to ingest food and fluids and adequacy of diet to support involution and lactation.
13. Assess ambulation, rest and exercise patterns, and ability to perform activities of daily living.
14. Assess peripheral circulation, noting varicosities, edema, and symmetry of size and shape, temperature, color, and range of motion. Note particularly signs of thrombophlebitis and positive Homan's sign.
15. Assess psychosocial adaptation, including:
    a.  Signs and symptoms of postpartum "blues," such as crying, despondency, loss of appetite, poor concentration, difficulty sleeping, anxiety.
    b.  Evaluate integration of the newborn into the family.
    c.  Observe interactions of the new mother and other family members with the newborn.

**B.  Nursing diagnoses**
1.  Anxiety
2.  Body Image Disturbance
3.  Constipation
4.  Risk for Infection
5.  Risk for Injury
6.  Knowledge Deficit
7.  Pain
8.  Altered Parenting
9.  Altered Role Performance
10. Self Care Deficit
11. Sexual Dysfunction
12. Altered Patterns of Urinary Elimination

**C.  Planning and implementation**
1.  Teach the new mother aspects of self-care and newborn care.
2.  Observe the new mother providing care for her newborn.
3.  **Report and record increased pulse rate, decreased blood pressure, and elevated temperature.**

4. Gently massage the fundus if boggy; express clots from the fundus as indicated.

5. **Apply ice or cold therapy to the episiotomy or lacerations immediately after delivery to decrease edema and provide anesthesia; thereafter, apply moist or dry heat therapy to promote comfort and healing.**

6. Apply anesthetic sprays, ointments, or witch hazel pads to the perineum to promote comfort; administer analgesia as ordered and indicated; offer sitz baths as needed.

7. Instruct the client on sitting properly to relieve pain: squeeze buttocks together and contract pelvic floor muscles before sitting. Also instruct her to wear perineal pads loosely and to lie in Sims' position.

8. Instruct the client to clean her breasts daily, with clean water if breast-feeding and with soap and water if bottle-feeding, and to wear a well-fitted brassiere.

9. Treat breast pain of bottle-feeding client with analgesics and ice packs.

10. Assist with breast-feeding as needed; explain mechanisms involved in lactation, breast care, positioning of client and newborn, and nursing techniques.

11. Offer the opportunity to void within first 4 to 8 hours after delivery and every 2 to 3 hours thereafter. If necessary, help stimulate urination by running water, placing her hands in warm water, giving warm beverage, providing privacy and support, or pouring warm water over the vulva.

12. Demonstrate how to clean the perineum after each voiding and defecation, wiping from front to back, and then how to wash hands and apply a perineal pad from front to back.

13. Provide adequate dietary fiber and fluids to promote bowel movements; if necessary, administer stool softeners, laxatives, suppositories, or enemas. Teach the importance of adequate fluid intake, exercise, proper diet, and a regular defecation time.

14. Ensure healthful nutrition and fluid intake.

15. Support the client's attempts at ambulation and exercise; explain the advantages of early ambulation and regular exercise in preventing complications and strengthening muscles of the back, pelvic floor, and abdomen.

16. Instruct the client to avoid garters or constricting clothing that can impair circulation.

17. During hospitalization, limit visitors, and adjust routine to enable adequate rest.

18. Permit the client to shower as soon as she can ambulate and to

take tub baths, if desired, after 2 weeks. Recommend a daily shower to promote comfort and a sense of well-being.

19. Provide emotional and psychological support during the transition to parenthood, including:
    a. Encouraging the mother to hold and explore her newborn
    b. Facilitating visitation by partner and others
    c. Providing time for parent–newborn contact, as indicated by the mother's and newborn's condition
    d. Explaining postpartum hormonal changes and how they can affect emotions and mood
    e. Demonstrating newborn care and safety measures
    f. Providing analgesia and position changes for comfort and promoting adequate rest; stressing the need for adequate rest to enhance coping ability
    g. Discussing expected newborn developmental milestones and expected maternal physical and psychological changes in the postpartum period
    h. Discussing resumption of sexual activity and planning birth control, if desired (Typically, intercourse can be safely resumed after 3 weeks; other forms of sexual expression need not be affected.)
    i. Explaining the newborn's need to be touched, held, and spoken to often; discussing the newborn's responses to various stimuli
    j. Allowing the new parents to express feelings and concerns

20. Advise the client to schedule a 4- to 6-week check-up to assess her general physical condition, progress of involution, and family adaptation to the newborn.

**D. Evaluation**

1. During the immediate postpartum period:
    a. The client exhibits normal uterine involution.
    b. Vital signs, weight, and healing of episiotomy are within accepted parameters.
    c. The client requests and tolerates food and fluids.
    d. The client empties bladder as needed.
    e. The client rests between procedures and observations.
    f. The client holds and explores newborn.

2. During postpartum hospitalization:
    a. Vital signs, weight, breasts, involutional process, and healing of episiotomy are within expected parameters.
    b. The client maintains bowel and bladder elimination.
    c. The client performs breast and perineal care.
    d. The client rests and sleeps.

      e.    The client verbalizes correct self-care and newborn care.

**3.**    In preparation for discharge:
    a.    The client demonstrates satisfactory newborn care ability.
    b.    The client verbalizes the importance of follow-up care for herself and her newborn.
    c.    The client knows how to contact primary physician, obstetrician, pediatrician, midwife, primary nurse.
    d.    The client expresses understanding of psychosocial needs of the newborn and parent–sibling–family interaction.
    e.    The couple verbalizes understanding of changes in sexual response, when they can safely resume intercourse, and the use of contraception.

**4.**    Findings at the routine postpartum check-up:
    a.    Weight, breast changes, involutional process, and healing of episiotomy are within expected parameters.
    b.    The client's reproductive organs return to near prepregnant condition.
    c.    The family demonstrates positive adaptation and function.
    d.    The client uses her preferred contraceptive method.

## Bibliography

Bobak, I. M., & Jensen, M. D. (1993). *Maternity and gynecologic care: The nurse and the family* (5th ed.). St. Louis: C.V. Mosby.

May, K. A., & Mahlmeister, L. R. (1994). *Maternal and neonatal nursing: Family-centered care* (3rd ed.). Philadelphia: J.B. Lippincott.

Olds, S. B., London, M. L., & Ladewig, P. W. (1992). *Maternal-newborn nursing: A family centered approach* (4th ed.). Menlo Park, CA: Addison-Wesley.

Reeder, S. J., Martin, L. L., & Koniak, D. (1992). *Maternity nursing: Family newborn, and women's health care* (17th ed.). Philadelphia: J.B. Lippincott.

# STUDY QUESTIONS

1. From the following, select the best definition of postpartum care:
   a. It is the time to prevent or minimize postpartum complications and anxiety.
   b. It is the time to provide effective discharge planning and referral for follow-up care.
   c. It is the time for medical and nursing personnel to provide sensitive professional care.
   d. It is the time for medical and nursing care to be given to the client from delivery to nonpregnant status.

2. Many postpartum biophysical changes take place soon after delivery. Which of the following statements is true about the uterus?
   a. The uterus contracts firmly, reducing its size by more than half; it remains this size for about 2 days and then becomes smaller and descends about one finger breadth daily.
   b. The uterus contracts firmly, reducing its size two and one-half times; it remains this size for several days and then shrinks as it descends five finger breadths per day.
   c. At 15 to 20 postpartum days, the uterus cannot be palpated abdominally. It returns to its nonpregnant size by 8 postpartum weeks.
   d. At 4 to 5 postpartum days, the uterus cannot be palpated abdominally. It returns to its nonpregnant size by 4 to 6 postpartum weeks.

3. Which of the following statements is true about breast-related changes in the early postpartum period?
   a. Estrogen and progesterone levels and secretion of prolactin rapidly increase.
   b. Colostrum is present by 2 to 3 postpartum days, and this eventually changes to breast milk.
   c. Estrogen and progesterone levels drop rapidly with the increase in prolactin secretion.
   d. The breasts become larger and firmer immediately so that the newborn will receive sufficient breast milk.

4. Why is it important to measure urine output for several days after delivery?
   a. A full bladder will displace the uterus and may cause postpartum hemorrhage.
   b. A full bladder will prolapse, causing a great deal of discomfort for the new mother.
   c. A full bladder will cause diaphoresis and therefore discomfort and pain.
   d. A full bladder will rupture during palpation of the uterine fundus after delivery.

5. The postpartum period represents a time of emotional stress for the new mother. Of the following, which factor most influences the new mother's successful transition to parenthood?
   a. Early discharge, which offers the mother and newborn an opportunity to attain needed rest and sleep at home
   b. The need of both parents to know that everything is okay and that no problems will occur
   c. The new mother having full emotional support of family and friends and being emotionally ready for parenthood
   d. The new mother understanding the signs and symptoms of postpartum "blues" and being able to deal with them

6. According to Rubin, in which period would the new mother frequently review her labor and delivery experience?
   a. During the postpartum depression period
   b. During the letting-go period
   c. During the taking-hold period
   d. During the taking-in period

7. Which of the following groups of signs and symptoms are the most representative of postpartum "blues"?
   a. Crying, loss of appetite, constipation, abdominal pain, and anxiety
   b. Crying, despondency, loss of appetite, difficulty sleeping, and anxiety
   c. Crying, increased appetite, urinary retention, anxiety, and fear of the unknown
   d. Crying, despondency, poor concentration, constipation, diarrhea, and anxiety

8. A client is visiting the clinic 2 weeks after delivery of her first child. While talking with the nurse, she asks, "When can John and I have sex?" Which response by the nurse would be the most appropriate?

   a. "It's okay now. I'm surprised John has been able to wait this long."
   b. "Are you breast-feeding or bottle feeding? That will make a difference."
   c. "Typically, intercourse can be safely resumed 3 weeks after delivery."
   d. "Why do you ask? Don't you get enough satisfaction from other forms of sexual expression?"

9. During this same visit to the clinic, the client asks whether her current vaginal discharge is normal. The nurse should know that at this time the client
   a. should have lochia alba
   b. should have lochia serosa
   c. should have lochia rubra
   d. should have lochia sanguineous

For additional questions, see
*Lippincott's Self-Study Series* Software
Available at your bookstore

# ANSWER KEY

1. **Correct response: d**

   Postpartum care refers to the medical and nursing care given to a client from the time of delivery until her body returns to its nonpregnant state.

   **a, b, and c.** All are possibilities, but they are not true definitions.

   *Knowledge/Safe Care/NA*

2. **Correct response: a**

   The uterus contracts firmly, reducing its size by more than half; it remains this size for about 2 days and then decreases in size (involution) and descends about one finger breadth per day.

   **b, c, and d.** These are incorrect answers.

   *Knowledge/Physiologic/Implementation*

3. **Correct response: c**

   Postpartum breast changes include rapid drop in estrogen and progesterone levels with an increase in secretion of prolactin after delivery.

   **a, b, and d.** All are incorrect answers.

   *Knowledge/Safe Care/NA*

4. **Correct response: a**

   A full bladder will displace the uterus and can cause postpartum hemorrhage; bladder distention can lead to urinary retention.

   **b and c.** These also may happen early postpartum but are not of major concern.

   **d.** This is an incorrect answer.

   *Knowledge/Safe Care/Assessment*

5. **Correct response: c**

   The postpartum period represents a time of emotional stress for the new mother, made even more difficult by the tremendous physiologic changes that occur. One of the factors influencing successful transition to parenthood is response and support of family and friends.

   **a and b** These are incorrect and

should not be used in this type of setting.

   **d.** Understanding is a difficult concept and therefore not measurable.

*Application/Safe Care/Evaluation*

6. **Correct response: d**

   According to Rubin, during the taking-in period, the new mother may review her labor and delivery experience frequently.

   **a, b, and c.** These are incorrect answers.

*Comprehension/Psychosocial/Implementation*

7. **Correct response: b**

   The group of postpartum signs and symptoms most characteristic of postpartum "blues" includes crying, despondency, loss of appetite, poor concentration, difficulty sleeping, and anxiety.

   **a, c, and d.** These may occur during the postpartum period, but together they do not constitute the syndrome known as the "blues."

*Comprehension/Psychosocial/Evaluation*

8. **Correct response: c**

   When questions related to the resumption of sexual activity arise, the best response would be that typically, intercourse can be safely resumed after 3 weeks; other forms of sexual expression need not be affected.

   **b.** Although the newborn feeding method may affect sexual desire, it has no effect on the time when sexual relations can safely resume.

   **a and d.** These are unprofessional answers.

*Application/Safe Care/Evaluation*

9. **Correct response: a**

   Lochia alba is seen 1 to 3 weeks postpartum.

b. Lochia serosa is seen 5 to 7 postpartum days.
c. Lochia rubra is seen 1 to 3 postpartum days.

d. This is an incorrect response.

*Comprehension/Safe Care/
Implementation*

# Newborn Care

*11*

## I. Overview

### A. Essential concepts

1. In the postpartum period, the newborn experiences complex biophysiologic and behavioral changes resulting from the transition to extrauterine life.

2. Nursing care of the newborn is based on knowledge of these changes and of the newborn's impact on the family unit.

3. The first few hours after birth represent a critical adjustment period for the newborn. In most settings, the nurse provides direct care to the newborn immediately after birth.

4. After the transition period, the nurse continues to evaluate the newborn at periodic intervals and to adjust nursing care plans according to ongoing findings.

5. The nurse must skillfully balance the family's need for privacy with the need to monitor the newborn's transition to extrauterine life.

**B. Goals of newborn care**

1. Initial postpartum period
   a. To establish and maintain an airway and support respirations
   b. To maintain warmth and prevent hypothermia
   c. To ensure safety and prevent injury or infection
   d. To identify actual or potential problems that may require immediate attention

2. Continuing care
   a. To continue protecting from injury or infection and identifying actual or potential problems that could require attention
   b. To facilitate development of a close parent–newborn relationship
   c. To provide parents with information about newborn care
   d. To assist parents in developing healthy attitudes about childrearing practices

**C. Factors affecting newborn adaptation**

1. Antepartum experiences of mother and newborn (eg, exposure to toxic substances, parental attitude toward childbearing and childrearing)
2. Intrapartum experiences of mother and newborn (eg, length of labor, type of intrapartum analgesia or anesthesia)
3. Newborn's physiologic capacity to make the transition to extrauterine life
4. Ability of health care providers to assess and respond appropriately in the event of problems

**D. Nursing responsibilities**

1. To support the newborn's physiologic adaptation to extrauterine life
2. To prevent or minimize potential complications
3. To facilitate parent–newborn interaction

**II. Transition to extrauterine life**

**A. Essential concepts**

1. Immediate initiation of respiration and changes in the circulatory patterns are essential for extrauterine life.
2. Within 24 hours after birth, the newborn's renal, gastrointestinal (GI), hematologic, metabolic, and neurologic systems must function sufficiently for progression to and maintenance of extrauterine life.

**B.** **Transition period**

1. This is a phase of instability during the first 6 to 8 hours of life through which all newborns pass, regardless of gestational age or nature of labor and delivery.

2. In the first period of reactivity (immediately after birth), respiration is rapid (may reach 80 per minute), and transient nostril flaring, retractions, and grunting may occur. The heart rate may reach 180 beats/min during the first few minutes of life.

3. Following this initial response, the newborn becomes quiet, relaxes, and falls asleep; this first sleep (known as the sleep phase) occurs within 2 hours of birth and lasts from a few minutes to several hours.

4. The second period of reactivity, starting when the newborn awakes, is marked by hyperresponsiveness to stimuli, skin color changes from pink to slightly cyanotic, and rapid heart rate.

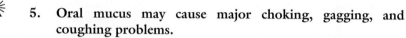

5. **Oral mucus may cause major choking, gagging, and coughing problems.**

**C.** **Respiratory adaptation**

1. Initial respirations are triggered by physical, sensory, and chemical factors:

   a. Physical factors: the effort required to expand the lungs and fill the collapsed alveoli (eg, change in pressure gradients)

   b. Sensory factors: temperature, noise, light, sound; drop in temperature thought to be the most important

   c. Chemical factors: changes in the blood (decreased $O_2$ level, increased $CO_2$ level, decreased pH) as a result of the transitory asphyxia during delivery

2. Newborn respiratory rate ranges between 30 and 60 breaths per minute.

3. Oral mucous secretions may cause the newborn to cough and gag, especially during first 12 to 18 hours.

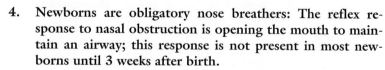

4. **Newborns are obligatory nose breathers: The reflex response to nasal obstruction is opening the mouth to maintain an airway; this response is not present in most newborns until 3 weeks after birth.**

**D.** **Cardiovascular adaptation**

1. Various anatomic changes take place after birth; some are immediate, others occur with time (Table 11-1).

2. Peripheral circulation is sluggish, causing acrocyanosis (cyanosis of the hands and feet and around the mouth).

3. Pulse rate is 120 to 160 beats/min while awake and 100 beats/min while asleep.

TABLE 11–1.
Changes in Fetal Circulation at Birth

| STRUCTURE | BEFORE BIRTH | AFTER BIRTH |
| --- | --- | --- |
| Umbilical vein | Brings arterial blood to liver and heart | Obliterated; becomes round ligament of liver |
| Umbilical arteries | Bring arteriovenous blood to placenta | Obliterated; become vesical ligaments on anterior abdominal wall |
| Ductus venosus | Shunts arterial blood into inferior vena cava | Obliterated; becomes ligamentum venosum |
| Ductus arteriosus | Shunts arterial and some venous blood from pulmonary artery to aorta | Obliterated; becomes ligamentum arteriosum |
| Foramen ovale | Connects right and left auricles (atria) | Obliterated usually; at times open |
| Lungs | Contain no air and very little blood; filled with fluid | Filled with air and well supplied with blood |
| Pulmonary arteries | Bring little blood to lungs | Bring much blood to lungs |
| Aorta | Receives blood from both ventricles | Receives blood only from left ventricle |
| Inferior vena cava | Brings venous blood from body and arterial blood from placenta | Brings blood only to right auricle |

4. Blood pressure averages 80/46 mm Hg and varies with size and activity of newborn.

5. See Table 11-2 for normal newborn hematologic values.

E. **Thermoregulation and metabolic changes**

1. The newborn's temperature may drop several degrees after delivery, because the external environment is cooler than the intrauterine environment.

2. A limited supply of subcutaneous fat and a large skin surface area in relation to body weight predispose the newborn to heat transfer with the environment.

3. Rapid heat loss in a cool environment occurs by conduction, convection, radiation, and evaporation.

4. **Cold stress (hypothermia) in the newborn, with its associated metabolic acidosis, can be lethal even for a vigorous, full-term newborn.**

F. **Neurologic adaptation**

1. The newborn's neurologic system is not fully developed anatomically or physiologically.

2. The newborn exhibits uncoordinated movements, labile temperature regulation, poor control over musculature, easy startling, and tremors of the extremities.

3. Neonatal development is rapid; as the newborn grows, more

TABLE 11–2.
Neonatal Blood Values

| PARAMETER | NORMAL RANGE |
|---|---|
| Hemoglobin | 15–20 g/dL |
| Red blood cells | 5.0–7.5 million/mm³ |
| Hematocrit | 43%–61% |
| White blood cells (WBCs) | 10,000–30,000/mm³ |
| Neutrophils | 40%–80% |
| Eosinophils | 2%–3% |
| Lymphocytes | 3%–10% |
| Monocytes | 6%–10% |
| Immature WBCs | 3%–10% |
| Platelets | 100,000–280,000/mm³ |
| Reticulocytes | 3%–6% |
| Blood volume | Early cord clamping: 78 mL/kg<br>Late cord clamping: 98.6 mL/kg<br>Third day after early cord clamping: 82.3 mL/kg<br>Third day after late cord clamping: 92.6 mL/kg |

complex patterns of behavior (eg, head control, smiling, and purposeful reaching) will develop.

4. Newborn reflexes are important indicators of normal development (Table 11-3).

**G. Gastrointestinal adaptation**

1. Digestive enzymes are active at birth and can support extrauterine life by 36 to 38 weeks' gestation.

2. The necessary muscular and reflex developments for transporting food are present at birth.

3. Digestion of protein and carbohydrates is readily accomplished; fat digestion and absorption are poor due to the inadequacy of pancreatic enzymes and lipase.

4. Salivary glands are immature at birth; little saliva is manufactured until 3 months.

 5. **Meconium, which is greenish black, viscous, and contains occult blood, is excreted within 24 hours in 90% of normal newborns.**

6. Wide variations occur among newborns regarding interest in food, symptoms of hunger, and amount of food ingested at any one sitting.

7. Some newborns nurse immediately when put to the breast; others take up to 48 hours for effective feeding.

8. Random hand-to-mouth movement and finger sucking have

TABLE 11-3.
Newborn Reflexes

| REFLEX | NORMAL RESPONSE | ABNORMAL RESPONSE |
|---|---|---|
| Rooting and sucking | Newborn turns head in direction of stimulus, opens mouth, and begins to suck when cheek, lip, or corner of mouth is touched with finger or nipple. | Weak or no response occurs with prematurity, neurologic deficit or injury, or central nervous system (CNS) depressions secondary to maternal drug ingestion (eg, narcotics). |
| Swallowing | Newborn swallows in coordination with sucking when fluid is placed on back of tongue. | Gagging, coughing, or regurgitation of fluid may occur; possibly associated with cyanosis secondary to prematurity, neurologic deficit, or injury; typically seen after laryngoscopy. |
| Extrusion | Newborn pushes tongue outward when tip of tongue is touched with finger or nipple. | Continuous extrusion of tongue or repetitive tongue thrusting occurs with CNS anomalies and seizures. |
| Moro | Bilateral symmetrical extension and abduction of all extremities, with thumb and forefinger forming characteristic "c," are followed by adduction of extremities and return to relaxed flexion when newborn's position changes suddenly or when newborn is placed on back on flat surface. | Asymmetrical response is seen with peripheral nerve injury (brachial plexus) or fracture of clavicle or long bone of arm or leg. No response occurs in cases of severe CNS injury. |
| Stepping | Newborn will step with one foot and then the other in walking motion when one foot is touched to flat surface. | Asymmetrical response is seen with CNS or peripheral nerve injury or fracture of long bone of leg. |
| Prone crawl | Newborn will attempt to crawl forward with both arms and legs when placed on abdomen on flat surface. | Asymmetrical response is seen with CNS or peripheral nerve injury or fracture of long bone. |
| Tonic neck "fencing" | Extremities on side to which head is turned will extend, and opposite extremities will flex when newborn's head is turned to one side while resting. Response may be absent or incomplete immediately after birth. | Persistent response after 4th month may indicate neurologic injury. Persistent absence seen in CNS injury and neurologic disorders. |
| Startle | Newborn abducts and flexes all extremities and may begin to cry when exposed to sudden movement or loud noise. | Absence of response may indicate neurologic deficit or injury. Complete and consistent absence of response to loud noises may indicate deafness. Response may be absent or diminished during deep sleep. |
| Crossed extension | Newborn's opposite leg will flex and then extend rapidly as if trying to deflect stimulus to other foot when placed in supine position; newborn will extend one leg in response to stimulus on bottom of foot. | Weak or absent response is seen with peripheral nerve injury or fracture of long bone. |
| Glabellar "blink" | Newborn will blink with first 4 or 5 taps to bridge of nose when eyes are open. | Persistent blinking and failure to habituate suggest neurologic deficit. |

(continued)

TABLE 11-3. (continued)

| REFLEX | NORMAL RESPONSE | ABNORMAL RESPONSE |
| --- | --- | --- |
| Palmar grasp | Newborn's finger will curl around object and hold on momentarily when finger is placed in palm of newborn's hand. | Response is diminished in prematurity. Asymmetry occurs with peripheral nerve damage (brachial plexus) or fracture of humerus. No response occurs with severe neurologic deficit. |
| Plantar grasp | Newborn's toes will curl downward when a finger is placed against the base of the toes. | Diminished response occurs with prematurity. No response occurs with severe neurologic deficit. |
| Babinski | Newborn's toes will hyperextend and fan apart from dorsiflexion of big toe when one side of foot is stroked upward from heel and across ball of foot. | No response occurs with CNS deficit. |

Adapted from May, K. A., & Mahlmeister. L. R. (1994). *Maternal and neonatal nursing: Family-centered care* (3rd ed.). Philadelphia: J.B. Lippincott.

been observed in utero; these actions are well developed at birth and are intensified with hunger.

**H. Kidney adaptation**

1. Glomerular filtration rate is relatively low at birth due to inadequate surface area of the glomerular capillaries.
2. Although these limitations do not compromise the healthy newborn, they do restrict the capacity of the newborn to respond to stressors.
3. Decreased ability to excrete drugs and excessive fluid loss can rapidly lead to acidosis and fluid imbalances.

4. **Most newborns void in the first 24 hours after birth and two to six times per day for the first 1 to 2 days; thereafter, they void 5 to 20 times in 24 hours.**

5. Urine may be cloudy from mucus and urate; a reddish stain ("brick dust") may be noticed on the diaper due to uric acid crystals.

**I. Hepatic adaptation**

1. During fetal life and to some degree after birth, the liver continues to aid in blood formation.
2. During the neonatal period, the liver produces substances essential for blood coagulation.

3. **Iron stores from the mother are sufficient to carry the**

newborn through the fifth month of extrauterine life; at this time, the newborn becomes susceptible to iron deficiency.

4. The liver also controls the amount of circulating unconjugated bilirubin, a pigment derived from the hemoglobin and released with the breakdown of red blood cells.

 5. **Unconjugated bilirubin can leave the vascular system and permeate other extravascular tissues (eg, the skin, sclera, oral mucous membranes), resulting in a yellow coloring termed *jaundice* or *icterus*.**

6. In protracted cold stress, anaerobic glycolysis occurs, resulting in increased acid production. Metabolic acidosis develops, and if there is a defect in respiratory function, respiratory acidosis also develops. Excessive fatty acids displace the bilirubin from the albumin-binding sites. The increased level of circulating unbound bilirubin that results increases the risk of kernicterus, even at serum bilirubin levels of 10 mg/dL or less.

**J.** **Immune system adaptation**

 1. **The newborn cannot limit an invading organism at the portal of entry.**

2. The immaturity of a number of protective systems significantly increases the risk of infection in the newborn period.

3. The inflammatory response is reduced qualitatively and quantitatively.

4. Phagocytosis is sluggish.

5. The acidity of the stomach and the production of pepsin and trypsin are not fully developed until 3 to 4 weeks of age.

6. Immunoglobulin A (IgA) is missing from the respiratory and urinary tracts; unless the newborn is breast-fed, IgA is absent from the GI tract as well.

 7. **Infection represents a leading cause of morbidity and mortality during the neonatal period.**

**III.** **Essentials of newborn assessment**

**A.** **Neonatal health history**

1. Comprehensive knowledge of the pregnancy, labor, and delivery is essential to understanding the significance of physical findings in the newborn.

2. A systematic approach helps ensure that pertinent data are not overlooked.

3. **Major categories of data**

   a. **Maternal prenatal history and care**

   b. **Maternal blood type and Rh factor, history of isoimmunization, antibody titers**

  c. **Maternal screening test results (eg, rubella titer, hepatitis antigen screen, venereal disease research laboratory,** *Chlamydia* **screen, gonorrhea cultures, herpes cultures, human immunodeficiency virus screen)**

  d. **Labor history: onset, length, complication**

  e. **Rupture of membranes: amount of fluid, presence of meconium, relationship to time of delivery**

  f. **Fetal monitoring record (eg, evidence of fetal distress, fetal scalp sampling, blood gas analysis results)**

  g. **Delivery history: length of second stage of labor, medications and anesthetic (amount and when administered)**

  h. **Postpartum history (eg, need for resuscitation, Apgar scores at 1 and 5 minutes)**

**B.** **Physical assessment**

 **1.** General appearance:

  a. Posture

  b. Skin: color, turgor, wrinkling, vernix caseosa, milia, lanugo, erythema toxicum, birthmarks

  c. Respiratory effort

 **2.** Vital sign and anthropometric assessment

  a. Respiratory rate: count breaths for 60 seconds before determining apical rate while newborn is quiet; normal rate is 30 to 60 breaths per minute.

  b. Heart rate: count apical rate for 60 seconds over the cardiac apex; normal rate is 120 to 160 beats/min.

  c. Temperature

   ▸ Take axillary temperature with thermometer held in axillary fold for 10 minutes; normal newborn temperature range is 36.4° to 37.2°C (97.5°–99°F).

   ▸ Take tympanic temperature with electronic sensor inserted in ear canal to measure temperature of blood circulating in internal carotid artery; accurate findings are available in seconds.

   ▸ Take rectal temperature (not preferred due to risk of trauma to rectal mucosa), if necessary, with thermometer inserted 0.25 to 0.5 in and with newborn's legs stabilized by nurse's hand.

  d. Weight: Weigh newborn at the same time each day before feeding; 95% of full-term newborns weigh 2,500 to 4,250 g.

  e. Length: Place newborn on flat surface and extend legs fully before measuring; average full-term length is 49.5 cm (19.5 in).

    f.   Head circumference: Measure around the fullest part of the occiput; average head circumference is 35.5 cm.

    g.   Chest circumference: Place measure over the nipples and across the lower border of the scapulae; average circumference is 33 cm, usually 2 to 3 cm smaller than head.

    h.   Blood pressure: though not routinely measured at birth, blood pressure assessed by Doppler ultrasound is the most accurate method in the newborn. It measures systolic, diastolic, and mean arterial pressures; average blood pressure at birth is 80/46 mm Hg.

**3.**   Detailed physical assessment involves:

    a.   Head and face

- Head size in proportion to body (normally about 25% of total body size)
- Presence of molding
- Symmetry of features
- Ocular hypertelorism (wide-spaced eyes—a distance of more than 3 cm between inner canthi of the eyes)

    b.   Fontanels

- Anterior fontanel (normally diamond shaped, 3–4 cm long and 2–3 cm wide; closes at 18 months)
- Posterior fontanel (normally triangle shaped, smaller than anterior; closes by 8–12 weeks)
- Tense, bulging fontanel (may indicate increased intracranial pressure)
- Sunken fontanel (characteristic of dehydration)

    c.   Eyes

- Color (usually appears blue or grey due to scleral thinness)
- Transient strabismus and nystagmus (common)
- Doll's eye phenomenon (may be seen when the head is turned and eye movements lag behind)

    d.   Nose and mouth

- Nasal patency, determined by closing the newborn's mouth and compressing one nostril at a time or by advancing a nasogastric tube
- Mucous secretions (if excessive, may indicate tracheoesophageal fistula)
- Precocious teeth, sucking calluses, and inclusion cysts (Epstein pearls) may be apparent

    e.   Ears and neck

- Ear pliability and flexibility (in a full-term newborn, normally soft and pliable and recoil readily when bent forward)

- ▶ Low-set ears, top of ear below level of the eyes' canthi (may indicate a chromosomal or organ abnormality)
- ▶ Hearing (normally well developed once the eustachian tube is cleared)
- ▶ Neck size (normally short with many thick folds)
- ▶ Neck webbing (associated with chromosomal abnormalities)

f.  Chest

- ▶ Contour and symmetry (normally round and symmetrical)
- ▶ Breast engorgement (may be evident 2 to 3 days after birth due to maternal hormones)
- ▶ Respirations (normally shallow, symmetrical, and synchronous with abdominal movement)
- ▶ Breath sounds: crackles (may be present during transitional period, representing fetal lung fluid and areas of atelectasis; should clear within several hours); rhonchi (indicating fluid, mucus, or meconium in the larger bronchi and possibly associated with life-threatening conditions, such as meconium aspiration)
- ▶ Heart sounds (about 90% of all murmurs transient and related to incomplete closure of the foramen ovale or ductus arteriosus)

g.  Abdomen

- ▶ Contour (normally rounded and protuberant due to weak abdominal musculature)
- ▶ Umbilical cord (normally appears white and gelatinous in the first few hours with two arteries and one vein apparent; begins to dry within a few hours)
- ▶ Shrunken, scaphoid appearance (indicates diaphragmatic hernia)
- ▶ Bowel sounds (normally audible when newborn is relaxed)

h.  Genitalia, female

- ▶ Labia minora (may have vernix and smegma in creases)
- ▶ Labia majora (normally cover the labia minora and clitoris)
- ▶ Clitoris (normally prominent)
- ▶ Vaginal discharge (may be present due to maternal hormones, called pseudomenstruation)
- ▶ Hymenal tag (normally present)

i.  Genitalia, male

- ▶ Scrotum (normally rugae present on scrotum and both testes descended into scrotum)
- ▶ Penis (Urinary meatus normally located at tip of glans; meatus on the dorsal surface, epispadias; on the ventral surface, hypospadias)

j.  Back and buttocks

▶ Spine (normally flat and round; tufts of hair or small indentations at the sacrum or base of the spine associated with spina bifida occulta)
▶ Patent anal opening

  k.  Upper extremities

▶ Flexion and movement (normally well flexed with symmetrical movement)
▶ Grasp reflex (normally present)
▶ Muscle tone and strength (partial or complete flaccidity of the arm may indicate trauma to brachial plexus)
▶ Brachial pulses (normally present)

  l.  Lower extremities

▶ Length and flexion (normally short, bowed, well flexed)
▶ Femoral and pedal pulses (normally present)

**C.  Neurologic assessment (newborn reflexes)**

  **1.**  Blink, cough, sneeze, and gag reflexes are present at birth and remain unchanged through adulthood.
  **2.**  Several reflexes are normally present at birth, reflecting neurologic immaturity; they disappear in the first year.
  **3.**  Sensory behaviors

  a.  Vision

▶ Can see objects about 6 to 8 in away
▶ Prefers black and white patterns
▶ Sensitive to light
▶ Can track parents with eyes
▶ Immature muscle coordination

  b.  Hearing: can detect sounds once eustachian tube clears
  c.  Taste

▶ Taste buds developed before birth
▶ Prefers sweet to bitter or sour tastes

  d.  Touch

▶ Can feel pressure, pain, and touch immediately or shortly after birth
▶ Sensitive to being cuddled

  e.  Smell

▶ After mucus and amniotic fluid are cleared from nasal passages, can differentiate pleasant from unpleasant odors
▶ Can distinguish mother's wet breast pad from another mother's at 1 week

**D.** Gestational age assessment

1. Systematic assessment of physical signs and neurologic traits helps estimate the newborn's gestational age.
2. To a large extent, degree of maturity at birth determines the ability of the newborn to survive.
3. **Determining gestational age provides information about system maturity and guides assessment of potential complications.**

**E.** Assessment of behavioral capabilities

1. Individual personalities, behavioral characteristics, and temperament play an important role in the ultimate relationship the newborn will form with parents and others.
2. By their actions, newborns encourage or discourage attachment and caretaking activities.
3. Awareness of the newborn's unique behavioral responses is important if parents are to learn to react to their newborn in ways that promote health.
4. Brazelton and others have devised scales to evaluate newborn behavior.

**IV. Nursing management of the normal newborn (transition period)**

**A.** Assessment

1. Evaluate respiratory status; determine Apgar score at 1 and 5 minutes (see Chap. 9).
2. Assess general status: size (weight, length, head and chest circumference), gestational age, normality of body systems, vital signs.
3. Measure axillary temperature every 30 minutes until stable and every 4 hours thereafter.
4. Assess blood glucose level on admission to the transition nursery and as indicated thereafter.

**B.** Nursing diagnoses

1. Ineffective Airway Clearance
2. Risk for Infection
3. Altered Nutrition: Less than body requirements
4. Ineffective Thermoregulation

**C.** Planning and implementation

1. Maintain airway patency; assess frequently, and keep a bulb syringe in bassinet.
2. Maintain a neutral thermal environment by placing the newborn under a radiant warmer; monitor temperature continuously using skin sensor until stable. Delay bathing until temperature stabilizes; dry newborn well after bath and return to radiant warmer until temperature is again stable.

3. Protect from infection: Use aseptic technique and administer prophylactic ophthalmic antibiotics.
4. Prevent nosocomial infection by instituting the following measures:
   a. Scrupulous handwashing technique
   b. "Clean" dress code (ie, scrub attire when entering nursery and cover gowns as indicated)
   c. Pre-employment and annual staff physical examinations to identify organisms that might be transmitted to newborns
5. Protect from hypoglycemia: Observe for jitteriness, tremors, eye rolling, weakness, high-pitched cry, poor muscle tone; use standard glucose test; and report result to physician if values are less than 40 mg/dL. Feed newborn according to established protocol (eg, breast milk, glucose water, formula).
6. Support establishment of feeding pattern.
7. Support parent–newborn attachment.
8. Prepare for routine procedures (eg, identifying newborn, administering vitamin K, and circumcision).
9. Initiate a teaching plan, covering such issues as bathing, cord care, care of the uncircumcised male, circumcision care, diapering and dressing, dealing with crying, formula preparation and sterilization, feeding techniques, burping, elimination patterns, prevention and care of diaper rash, swaddling or wrapping, handling and carrying, temperature measurement, safety considerations, signs and symptoms of illness, administration of common medications (eg, vitamins, antipyretics), and clearing nasal passages with bulb syringe.
10. If indicated, remind the parents when to return for ambulatory laboratory studies (eg, phenylketonuria, bilirubin).

**D. Evaluation**
1. The newborn breathes without assistance, as evidenced by normal respirations between 30 and 60 breaths per minute within 2 hours of birth.
2. The newborn maintains stable temperature, as evidenced by axillary temperature of 36.4° to 37.2°C (97.5°–99°F) within 1 to 2 hours of birth.
3. The newborn demonstrates normal cardiac output, as evidenced by a regular heart rate of 120 to 160 beats/min within 2 hours of birth.
4. The newborn shows no evidence of injury or infection.
5. The newborn begins to take nourishment within 4 to 8 hours of birth.
6. The mother demonstrates ability to feed the newborn by the time of discharge.

7. The newborn does not develop symptoms of hypoglycemia, or evident symptoms resolve without further complications within 12 to 24 hours.

8. The newborn and parents demonstrate interaction, as evidenced by touching, eye contact, and responsiveness to each other.

## V. Nursing management of the normal newborn (continuing care)

### A. Assessment

1. Review maternal, labor, delivery, and postpartum histories for pertinent or exceptional information.

2. Assess newborn's general status and gestational age, if indicated. Evaluate size, maturity, body systems, and vital signs, according to parameters established by standard assessment scales. These scales typically match measurements with gestational age.

   a. Size: Compare newborn's size (weight, length, and head circumference) with standards, such as those established by Lubchenko and colleagues. These models can be used to identify newborns with an excellent chance for normal growth or newborns at risk for various reasons. For example, they may be small at term or small for gestational age or out of proportion to other measurements (suggesting special problems, such as dwarfism or fused suture lines).

   b. Maturity: Physical and neuromuscular maturity may be estimated by using a standard, such as the Ballard assessment criteria. The Ballard scale assigns scores to 13 parameters, including neonatal postures and postural angles, and developmental hallmarks, such as plantar creases and genital characteristics. The total score reflects an assigned gestational age. For example, a score of 10 correlates with 28 gestational weeks, 15 with 30 weeks, 20 with 32 weeks, and so forth.

3. Evaluate fluid and caloric intake.

4. Assess elimination patterns (voiding within 24 hours, bowel movement within 24 hours).

5. Obtain and record daily weight; assess weight loss or weight gain.

### B. Nursing diagnoses

1. Constipation
2. Diarrhea
3. Fluid Volume Deficit
4. Altered Health Maintenance
5. Altered Nutrition: Less than body requirements
6. Risk for Infection

**C.** **Planning and implementation**

1. Because some newborns initially lose between 5% and 10% of birth weight, promote adequate hydration and nutrition (newborn nutritional needs: calories, 120 cal/kg per day; fluid, 140 to 160 mL/kg per day).
2. Promote normal elimination patterns.
3. Promote positive parent–newborn attachment.
4. Promote health maintenance (depending on the length of stay, discharge teaching is initiated on the unit and completed in the community during follow-up care of the family).
5. Recognize that discharge may occur as early as 6 hours after delivery, and plan teaching accordingly.
6. Arrange for ongoing assessment of the newborn's (and mother's) status (eg, home follow-up visits and parent education classes).

**D.** **Evaluation**

1. The newborn regains birth weight by 7 to 14 days after birth.
2. The newborn demonstrates urinary and bowel elimination patterns within normal limits for mode of feeding.
3. Parents demonstrate growing comfort and ease in handling newborn by the time of discharge.
4. The newborn continues to make physical and behavioral adaptations and is screened for congenital conditions, as appropriate, within the first week of life.

## Bibliography

Bobak, I. M., & Jensen, M. D. (1993). *Maternity and gynecologic care: The nurse and the family* (5th ed.). St. Louis: C.V. Mosby.

Gorrie, T. M., McKinney, E. S., & Murray, S. S. (1994). *Foundations of maternal newborn nursing*. Philadelphia: W.B. Saunders.

May, K. A., & Mahlmeister, L. R. (1994). *Maternal and neonatal nursing: Family-centered care* (3rd ed.). Philadelphia: J.B. Lippincott.

Olds, S. B., London, M. L., & Ladewig, P. W. (1992). *Maternal-newborn nursing: A family centered approach* (4th ed.). Menlo Park, CA: Addison-Wesley.

Reeder, S. J., Martin, L. L., & Koniak, D. (1992). *Maternity nursing: Family newborn, and women's health care* (17th ed.). Philadelphia: J.B. Lippincott.

# STUDY QUESTIONS

1. From the following, select a nursing goal of newborn care in the initial post-partum period.
   a. To facilitate development of a close parent–newborn relationship
   b. To assist parents in developing healthy attitudes about childrearing practices
   c. To identify actual or potential problems that may require immediate or emergency attention
   d. To provide the parents of the newborn with information about well-baby programs

2. Before birth, which of the following structures connects the right and left auricles of the heart?
   a. The umbilical vein
   b. The foramen ovale
   c. The ductus arteriosus
   d. The ductus venosus

3. After birth, which of the following structures receives blood only from the left ventricle?
   a. The aorta
   b. The inferior vena cava
   c. The pulmonary arteries
   d. The ductus arteriosus

4. During the initial respiratory adaptation period, many changes occur. Select the correct change that occurs during this period.
   a. Changes occur in the blood due to increased oxygen, decreased carbon dioxide, and decreased pH.
   b. The newborn's respiratory rate is rapid, and transient nasal flaring may be observed.
   c. The newborn respiratory rate is marked by hyperresponsiveness to stimuli.
   d. Changes occur in the blood due to decreased oxygen, increased carbon dioxide, and decreased pH.

5. Most newborns void in the first 24 hours after birth. Which of the following may cause a reddish stain on the diaper?
   a. Mucus and urate in the urine
   b. Uric acid crystals in the urine
   c. Bilirubin in the urine
   d. Excess iron in the urine

6. Select the *key concept* in regard to the newborn's immune system.
   a. Iron stores from the mother are sufficient to carry the newborn through the fifth month of extrauterine life.
   b. Unconjugated bilirubin can leave the vascular system and permeate other extravascular tisues.
   c. The newborn is unable to limit invading organisms at their point of entry.
   d. Most newborns void in the first 24 hours after birth and 5 to 20 times thereafter.

7. The heart rate of the newborn should be about
   a. 100 to 120 beats/min
   b. 80 to 100 beats/min
   c. 120 to 160 beats/min
   d. 120 to 140 beats/min

8. Which of the following is true regarding the fontanels of the newborn?
   a. There are two fontanels, the triangle-shaped anterior and the diamond-shaped posterior. Both close at 8 to 12 weeks.
   b. There are two fontanels. The anterior closes at 8 to 12 weeks, and the posterior closes at 18 months.
   c. There are two fontanels, the anterior and the posterior, both of which close at 18 months.
   d. There are two fontanels. The anterior closes at 18 months, and the posterior closes at 8 to 12 weeks.

9. Select the group of newborn reflexes below that are present at birth and remain unchanged through adulthood.
   a. The blink, cough, rooting, and gag reflexes

b. The blink, cough, sneeze, and gag reflexes

c. The rooting, sneeze, swallowing, and cough reflexes

d. The stepping, blink, cough, and sneeze reflexes

10. Which of the following best describes the Babinski reflex?

a. The newborn's toes will hyperextend and fan apart from dorsiflexion of the big toe when one side of foot is stroked upward from the heel and across the ball of the foot.

b. The newborn's toes will hyperextend and squeeze together from dorsiflexion of the big toe when one side of foot is stroked upward from the heel and across the ball of the foot.

c. The newborn's toes will hyperextend and fan apart from dorsiflexion of the big toe when one side of the foot is stroked across the ball of the foot and downward toward the heel.

d. The newborn's entire foot will pull away from the examiner's hand when the big toe is hyperextended and fan apart when one side of the foot is stroked upward from the heel and across the ball of the foot.

For additional questions, see
*Lippincott's Self-Study Series* Software
Available at your bookstore

# ANSWER KEY

1. **Correct Response: c**
One of the nursing goals of newborn care is to identify actual and potential problems that might require immediate attention.
**a, b, and d.** All are considered to be continuing care goals. All of these should be carried out only after the initial goals are met.
*Application/Health Promotion/Planning*

2. **Correct Response: b**
The foramen ovale is an opening between the right and left auricles (atria) that should close shortly after birth so the newborn will not have a murmur or mixed blood traveling through the vascular system.
**a, c, and d.** These are all incorrect answers.
*Comprehension/Physiologic/NA*

3. **Correct Response: a**
Before birth, the aorta carries blood from both of the ventricles. After birth, the aorta receives blood from the left ventricle.
**b, c, and d.** All are incorrect answers.
*Comprehension/Physiologic/NA*

4. **Correct Response: d**
Initial respirations are triggered by physical, sensory, and chemical factors. The chemical factors include the decreased oxygen level, increased carbon dioxide level, and a decrease in the pH as a result of the transitory asphyxia that occurs during delivery.
**a.** This is incorrect.
**b and c.** These are not chemical factors.
*Analysis/Physiologic/Implementation*

5. **Correct Response: b**
Uric acid crystals in the urine may produce the reddish "brick dust" stain on the diaper.
**a.** Mucus and urate do not produce a stain.

**c and d.** Bilirubin and iron are from hepatic adaptation.
*Analysis/Physiologic/Assessment*

6. **Correct Response: c**
The newborn cannot limit the invading organism at the port of entry.
**a, b, and d.** These are true of adaptations in other body systems.
*Application/Safe Care/Analysis*

7. **Correct Response: c**
The apical heart rate should be counted for 60 seconds over the cardiac apex while the newborn is quiet. The normal rate is between 120 and 160 beats/min.
**a, b, and d.** All are incorrect. These ranges may indicate actual or potential problems.
*Knowledge/Physiologic/NA*

8. **Correct Response: d**
There are two fontanels. The diamond-shaped anterior fontanel closes at 18 months. The triangular posterior fontanel closes by 8 to 12 weeks.
**a, b, and c.** All are incorrect.
*Knowledge/Safe Care/Assessment*

9. **Correct Response: b**
Blink, cough, sneeze, swallow, and gag reflexes are all present at birth and remain unchanged through adulthood.
**a, c, and d.** These groups of reflexes are all present at birth, but some reflexes, such as rooting and stepping, subside within the first year.
*Knowledge/Physiologic/Assessment*

10. **Correct Response: a**
The newborn's toes will hyperextend and fan apart from dorsiflexion of the big toe when one side of foot is stroked upward from the heel and across the ball of the foot.
**b, c, and d.** These variations of the classic Babinski reflex are incorrect; they would suggest actual or potential central nervous system deficits.
*Analysis/Physiologic/NA*

# Antepartum Complications

## 12

## I. Overview

### A. Essential concepts

1. Although most pregnancies progress to successful delivery without complications, various factors can alter the physiologic processes of pregnancy and compromise the well-being of the mother or the developing fetus.

 2. **These complications may occur at any time during pregnancy and can result from preexisting maternal medical problems or from the pregnancy itself.**

3. Significant complications of pregnancy include:
   a. Sponaneous abortion
   b. Gestational trophoblastic disease (hydatidiform mole)
   c. Ectopic pregnancy
   d. Incompetent cervix
   e. Hyperemesis gravidarum
   f. Anemia
   g. Placenta previa
   h. Abruptio placentae
   i. Pregnancy-induced hypertension (PIH)
   j. Gestational diabetes
   k. Hemolytic disease of the fetus and newborn

4. Maternal conditions that can significantly affect the fetus or the progress of pregnancy include diabetes mellitus, cardiac disease, hematologic disorders (eg, anemia, hemoglobinopathies), infections, sexually transmitted diseases, and substance abuse.

5. **Major goals of prenatal nursing are screening for and preventing complications and developing therapeutic interventions.**

6. Early and consistent prenatal care results in improved fetal and maternal outcome, regardless of complications that may occur.

**B.** **General nursing management of clients at risk**
1. Assessment: Evaluate each pregnancy to identify at-risk clients as early as possible.
2. Nursing diagnoses: In addition to the complication-specific diagnoses, the following nursing diagnoses are common to care of the at-risk antepartum client.
   a. Anxiety
   b. Ineffective Individual Coping
   c. Ineffective Family Coping: Compromised
   d. Altered Family Processes
   e. Fear
   f. Altered Role Performance
   g. Body Image Disturbance
   h. Knowledge Deficit
   i. Powerlessness
3. Planning and implementation: Begin intervening early to prevent or alleviate problems or potential problems.
4. Evaluation: The client and family experience an optimal birth event, having coped successfully with a preexisting or emergent complication of pregnancy.

**II. Spontaneous abortion**
   **A.** **Description: Spontaneous abortion is the expulsion of the fetus and other products of conception from the uterus before the fetus is viable.**
   **B.** **Etiology and pathophysiology**

   1. **Spontaneous abortion may result from unidentified natural causes or from fetal, placental, or maternal factors.**
   2. Fetal factors
      a. Defective embryologic development
      b. Faulty ovum implantation
      c. Rejection of the ovum by the endometrium
      d. Chromosomal abnormalities
   3. Placental factors
      a. Premature separation of the normally implanted placenta
      b. Abnormal placental implantation
      c. Abnormal platelet function
   4. Maternal factors
      a. Infection
      b. Severe malnutrition
      c. Reproductive system abnormalities (eg, incompetent cervix)
      d. Endocrine problems (eg, thyroid dysfunction)
      e. Trauma
      f. Drug ingestion

5.  Kinds of spontaneous abortions
   a.  Threatened: cramping and vaginal bleeding in early pregnancy with no cervical dilation. It may subside or an incomplete abortion may follow.
   b.  Imminent or inevitable: bleeding, cramping, and cervical dilation. Termination cannot be prevented.
   c.  Incomplete: expulsion of only part of the products of conception (placenta). Bleeding occurs with cervical dilation.
   d.  Complete: complete expulsion of all products of conception
   e.  Missed: early fetal intrauterine death without expulsion of the products of conception. The cervix is closed, and the client may report dark brown vaginal discharge. Pregnancy test findings are negative.
   f.  Habitual: spontaneous abortion of three or more consecutive pregnancies

**C.**  **Assessment findings**

  1.  **Common signs and symptoms of spontaneous abortion**
   a.  **Vaginal bleeding in the first 20 weeks of pregnancy**
   b.  **Complaints of cramping in lower abdomen**
   c.  **Fever, malaise, or other symptoms of infection**
   2.  The client and family may exhibit a grief reaction at the loss of pregnancy, such as crying, depression, sustained or prolonged social isolation, and withdrawal.

**D.**  **Nursing diagnoses**
   1.  Fluid Volume Deficit
   2.  Anticipatory Grieving
   3.  Dysfunctional Grieving
   4.  Risk for Infection

**E.**  **Planning and implementation**
   1.  Assess and record vital signs, bleeding, and cramping or pain.
   2.  Obtain history of previous pregnancies.
   3.  Offer emotional support and anticipatory guidance relative to expected recovery, need for rest, and delay of another pregnancy until the client fully recovers.
   4.  Suggest avoiding intercourse until after the next menses or using condoms when engaging in intercourse.
   5.  Recommend iron supplements and increased dietary iron as indicated to help prevent anemia.

  6.  **Prepare for RhoGAM administration to an Rh-negative mother, as prescribed.**
   7.  Measure and record intravenous fluids, vital signs, and labora-

tory test results in instances of heavy vaginal bleeding; prepare for surgery if indicated.

8. Offer emotional support because the client may experience guilt, grief, and loss.
9. Explain that in many cases, no cause is ever identified.
10. Describe self-care measures as appropriate.

F. **Evaluation**
   1. The client responds to teaching about diet, iron supplementation, and rest.
   2. The client and family demonstrate behaviors associated with normal grieving without signs of morbid grief reaction.
   3. The client remains free of infection.
   4. The client responds to iron supplementation by maintaining normal blood values.
   5. The client maintains fluid volume balance, as evidenced by normal vital signs and hydration status.

III. **Gestational trophoblastic disease (hydatidiform mole)**
   A. **Description: An alteration of early embryonic growth causing placental disruption, rapid proliferation of abnormal cells, and destruction of the embryo.**
   B. **Etiology and pathophysiology**
      1. A placental tumor that develops after pregnancy has occurred, a hydatidiform mole may be benign or malignant.
      2. The embryo dies and the trophoblastic cells continue to grow, forming an invasive tumor.
      3. It is characterized by proliferation of placental villi that become edematous and form grapelike clusters.
      4. Blood vessels are absent, as are a fetus and amniotic sac.
      5. Genetic abnormalities at the time of fertilization are thought to be responsible for trophoblastic disease.
   C. **Assessment findings**
      1. Signs and symptoms of gestational trophoblastic disease
         a. Severe nausea and vomiting
         b. PIH before 20 weeks' gestation
         c. Vaginal bleeding (may contain some of the edematous villi)
         d. Uterus larger than expected for the duration of the pregnancy
         e. Abdominal cramping from uterine distention
      2. Associated findings
         a. Abnormally high serum levels of human choronic gonadotropin (HCG)
         b. Characteristic appearance of molar growth on ultrasound tracing

**D.** **Nursing diagnoses**
1. Anxiety
2. Anticipatory Grief
3. Body Image Disturbance
4. Fear
5. Knowledge Deficit
6. Fluid Volume Deficit

**E.** **Planning and implementation**
1. Establish initial data base on admission.
2. Review pertinent history and history of this pregnancy.
3. Assist with the physical examination.
4. Assess the woman's feelings toward the pregnancy and her understanding of the problem.
5. Administer intravenous fluids as prescribed.

 6. **Prepare for suction curettage evacuation of the uterus. (Induction of labor with oxytocic agents or prostaglandins is not recommended because of the increased risk of hemorrhage.)**
7. Explain the need for frequent follow-up physical and pelvic examinations. Also explain that HCG levels should be monitored for 1 year.
8. Discuss the need to prevent pregnancy for at least 1 year after diagnosis and treatment.
9. Inform the client that oral birth control agents are not recommended because they suppress pituitary luteinizing hormone, which may interfere with serum HCG measurement.

 10. **Describe and emphasize signs and symptoms that must be reported (ie, irregular vaginal bleeding, persistent secretion from the breast, hemoptysis, and severe persistent headaches). These symptoms may indicate spread of the disease to other organs.**

**F.** **Evaluation**
1. The client responds to treatment.
2. The client verbalizes understanding of the importance of following the treatment plan.
3. The client keeps follow-up appointments to assess the possibility of recurrence of the problem or progression to choriocarcinoma.
4. The client practices safe, effective contraception.
5. The client is free of complications.

**IV.** **Ectopic pregnancy**

    **A.** Description: implantation of products of conception in a site other than the endometrium (eg, fallopian tube, ovary, cervix, peritoneal cavity)

    **B.** Etiology and pathophysiology

        **1.** Ectopic pregnancy can result from conditions that hinder ovum passage through the fallopian tube and into the uterine cavity, such as:

            a. Endosalpingitis

            b. Diverticula

            c. Tumors

            d. Adhesions from previous surgery

            e. Transmigration of the ovum from one ovary to the opposite fallopian tube

        **2.** Maternal prognosis is good with early diagnosis and prompt treatment, such as salpingostomy or tubal segmentation, or other therapies, such as methotrexate, which may preserve the tube but must meet several criteria (eg, before 6 weeks of pregnancy and before the fetal heart beats).

    **C.** Assessment findings

        **1.** Common clinical manifestations

            a. Dizziness, syncope (faintness)

            b. Sharp abdominal pain, referred shoulder pain

            c. Vaginal bleeding

            d. Adnexal mass and tenderness

        **2.** The client with ectopic pregnancy may report signs and symptoms of normal pregnancy or may have no symptoms at all.

        **3.** **Suspect ectopic pregnancy in a client whose history includes a missed menstrual period, spotting or pelvic pain, intrauterine device use, pelvic infections, or tubal surgery.**

        **4.** **Be alert for a ruptured fallopian tube, which can produce life-threatening complications, such as hemorrhage, shock, and peritonitis.**

    **D.** Nursing diagnoses

        **1.** Anxiety

        **2.** Anticipatory Grief

        **3.** Knowledge Deficit

        **4.** Pain

    **E.** Planning and implementation

        **1.** Assess vital signs, bleeding, and pain.

        **2.** Explain the condition, and describe self-care measures, which depend on the treatment.

        3.    Offer emotional support as the client grieves for her lost pregnancy.

**F. Evaluation**

        1.    The client remains free of complications.

        2.    The client verbalizes understanding of the condition.

        3.    The client exhibits functional grieving.

## V. Incompetent cervix

**A.** **Description: Characterized by painless dilation of the cervical os without contractions of the uterus, incompetent cervix usually occurs in the second or early third trimester (average, between 14 and 16 weeks).**

**B. Etiology and pathophysiology**

        1.    History of traumatic birth

        2.    Forceful dilatation and curettage

        3.    Client's mother treated with diethylstilbestrol (DES) when pregnant with the client

        4.    Congenitally short cervix

        5.    Uterine anomalies

        6.    Unknown etiology

**C. Assessment findings**

        1.    History of cervical trauma

        2.    Appreciable cervical dilation with prolapse of the membranes through the cervix without labor

        3.    History of repeated, spontaneous, second trimester terminations

        4.    Possibly spontaneous rupture of the membranes

**D. Nursing diagnoses**

        1.    Anxiety

        2.    Situational Low Self Esteem

        3.    Ineffective Individual Coping

        4.    Altered Family Process

        5.    Knowledge Deficit

        6.    Anticipatory Grief

**E. Planning and implementation**

        1.    Assess the client's feelings about herself and the pregnancy.

        2.    Explain incompetent cervix.

        3.    Evaluate the client's support systems.

        4.    Assess for appropriate coping responses.

        5.    Offer emotional support as needed.

        6.    Prepare for surgical intervention, such as cervical cerclage (suturing the cervix).

        7.    Administer tocolytic medications as prescribed.

        8.    Maintain activity restrictions as prescribed.

        9.    Demonstrate application of the uterine contraction monitor for home monitoring if required.

10. Discuss the need for vaginal rest (no intercourse or orgasm).
11. Describe problems that must be reported immediately (ie, signs of labor, rupture of membranes, signs of infection).

   **F.** **Evaluation**
   1. The client verbalizes her concerns and fears.
   2. The client demonstrates effective self-care behaviors to maintain the pregnancy.
   3. The client uses effective coping behaviors.
   4. The client verbalizes understanding of her condition and its treatment.
   5. The client complies with the treatment regimen.
   6. The client is free of further complications. If additional problems arise, she receives prompt and appropriate treatment.

**VI.** **Hyperemesis gravidarum**
   **A.** **Description: severe nausea and vomiting, leading to electrolyte, metabolic, and nutritional imbalances in the absence of other medical problems**
   **B.** **Etiology and pathophysiology**
   1. Some experts suspect that the rapidly increasing levels of HCG in early pregnancy induces emesis; however, this theory remains unproved.
   2. Continued vomiting results in dehydration and ultimately decreases the amount of blood and nutrients circulated to the developing fetus.
   3. Hospitalization may be required for severe symptoms when the client needs intravenous hydration and correction of metabolic imbalances.

   4. **Signs and symptoms occur during the first 16 weeks of pregnancy and are intractable.**
   **C.** **Assessment findings**
   1. Signs and symptoms of hyperemesis gravidarum
      a. Unremitting nausea and vomiting
      b. Vomitus initially containing undigested food, bile, and mucus; later, blood and material, resembling coffee grounds
      c. Weight loss
   2. Associated findings
      a. Pale, dry skin
      b. Subnormal or elevated temperature
      c. Rapid pulse
      d. Fetid, fruity breath odor from acidosis
      e. Central nervous system effects, such as confusion, delirium, headache, and lethargy, stupor, or coma

**D.** **Nursing diagnoses**
   1. Anxiety
   2. Fluid Volume Deficit
   3. Altered Nutrition: Less than body requirements

**E.** **Planning and implementation**
   1. Administer intravenous fluids as prescribed; they may be given on an ambulatory basis when dehydration is mild.
   2. Measure and record intake and output.
   3. Maintain a nonjudgmental atmosphere in which the client and family can express concerns and resolve some of their fears.

**F.** **Evaluation**
   1. The client responds to treatment; nausea and vomiting subside, and weight gain is maintained.
   2. The client keeps follow-up appointments to assess progress of pregnancy.

**VII.** **Anemia**

**A.** **Description: hemoglobin value of 10 g or less during the second and third trimesters**

**B.** **Etiology and pathophysiology**

   1. **Causes of anemia include nutritional deficiency (iron deficiency, megaloblastic anemia, which includes folic acid deficiency and $B_{12}$ deficiency), acute and chronic blood loss, and hemolysis (sickle cell anemia, thalassemia, G6PD).**
   2. Iron deficiency anemia is common during pregnancy, affecting 15% to 50% of pregnant women.
   3. Mild anemia (hemoglobin value of 11 g) poses no threat but is an indication of a less than optimal nutritional state.
   4. Maternal morbidity is uncommon unless hemoglobin level drops below 6 g.
   5. More subtle complications (delayed wound healing, infection, postpartum hemorrhage) are associated with less severe reductions in hemoglobin level.
   6. Hemoglobinopathies, such as thalassemia, sickle cell disease, and G6PD, lead to anemia by causing hemolysis or increased destruction of red blood cells.
   7. Pseudoanemia of pregnancy may result from hypervolemia.

**C.** **Assessment findings**
   1. **Review the health history, physical findings, and current symptoms.**
   2. Anticipate findings of urinary tract infection, chest colds, and pulmonary congestion. These should be identified early and treated appropriately.
   3. In clients with a hemoglobin level below 10.5 g, expect complaints of excessive fatigue, headache, and tachycardia.

    4.   Observe for brittle fingernails, cheilosis (severely chapped lips), or a smooth, red, shiny tongue. These are signs of severe iron deficiency anemia.

**D.**  **Nursing diagnoses**

    1.   Ineffective Individual or Family Coping

    2.   Knowledge Deficit

    3.   Altered Nutrition: Less than body requirements

    4.   Constipation

**E.**  **Planning and implementation**

    1.   Discuss using iron supplements and increasing dietary sources of iron as indicated.

    2.   Describe self-care measures that may prevent complications, but also describe signs and symptoms of complications to report to the nurse or physician.

    3.   Prepare for blood typing and cross-matching and for administering packed red blood cells during labor if the client has severe anemia.

    **4.**   **In a client who has thalassemia or who carries the trait, provide support, especially if the woman has just learned that she is a carrier. Also assess for signs of infection throughout the pregnancy.**

    5.   In a pregnant client with sickle cell disease, assess iron and folate stores and reticulocyte counts; complete screening for hemolysis; provide dietary counseling and folic acid supplements; and observe for signs of infection.

    6.   In a pregnant client with G6PD, provide iron and folic acid supplementation and nutrition counseling, and explain the need to avoid oxidizing drugs.

**F.**  **Evaluation**

    1.   The client and family verbalize understanding of anemia.

    2.   The client complies with the treatment regimen.

    3.   The client maintains adequate nutrition.

    4.   Hemoglobin levels respond to treatment, and pregnancy continues without related undesired events.

**VIII.**  **Placenta previa**

**A.**  **Description: In placenta previa, the placenta implants in the lower uterine segment, causing painless bleeding in the third trimester of pregnancy (about 30 weeks).**

**B.**  **Etiology and pathophysiology**

    1.   Pathologic process seems to be related to the conditions that alter the normal function of the uterine decidua and its vascularization.

    2.   Predisposing factors

    a. Multiparity (80% of affected clients are multiparous)

    b. Advanced maternal age (older than 35 years in 33% of cases)

    c. Multiple gestation

    d. Previous cesarean birth

    e. Uterine incisions

    f. Prior placenta previa (incidence is 12 times greater in women with previous placenta previa)

  **3.** Bleeding, which results from tearing of the placental villi from the uterine wall as the lower uterine segment contracts and dilates, can be slight or profuse.

  **4.** Incidence is one in 300 deliveries.

  **5.** Placenta previa may be classified as:

    a. Total: Placenta completely covers the internal os.

    b. Partial: Placenta partially covers the internal os.

    c. Low lying or low implantation: Placenta reaches the area of the internal os.

**C.** **Assessment findings**

  **1.** Signs and symptoms of placenta previa

    a. Bright red, painless vaginal bleeding

    b. Soft, nontender abdomen; relaxes between contractions

    c. Fetal heart rate (FHR) stable and within normal limits

  **2.** Suspicion of placenta previa may be confirmed by transabdominal ultrasonography.

  **3.** **In cases of suspected placenta previa, vaginal examination is delayed until ultrasound results are available and the client is moved to the operating room for what is termed a double-setup procedure. The operating room is needed because the examination can cause further tearing of the villi and profuse bleeding.**

**D.** **Nursing diagnoses**

  **1.** Activity Intolerance

  **2.** Fear

  **3.** Anticipatory Grieving

  **4.** Risk for Infection

  **5.** Decreased Cardiac Output

  **6.** Fluid Volume Deficit

  **7.** Altered Family Processes

**E.** **Planning and implementation**

  **1.** Take and record vital signs, assess bleeding, and maintain pad count.

  **2.** Observe for shock (rapid pulse, pallor, cold moist skin, drop in blood pressure).

  **3.** Monitor FHR.

4. Enforce strict bed rest to minimize risk to the fetus.
5. Observe for additional bleeding episodes.
6. Offer emotional support to facilitate the grieving process if needed.
7. Explain the condition and management options.
8. Prepare for ambulation and discharge (may be within 48 hours of last bleeding episode).
9. Discuss the need to have transportation to the hospital available at all times.

10. **Instruct client to return to the hospital if bleeding recurs and to avoid intercourse until after the birth.**

**F.** Evaluation
1. The client demonstrates compliance with prescribed activity limitations.
2. The client and family exhibit functional grieving.
3. The client remains free from complications.
4. The client gives birth to a healthy newborn at or near term.

## IX. Abruptio placentae

**A.** **Description: premature separation of a normally implanted placenta during the second half of pregnancy, typically with severe hemorrhage**

**B.** Etiology and pathophysiology
1. The cause of abruptio placentae is unknown.
2. Risk factors
   a. Uterine anomalies
   b. Multiparity
   c. PIH
   d. Previous cesarean delivery
   e. Renal or vascular disease
   f. Trauma to abdomen
   g. Previous third-trimester bleeding
   h. Abnormally large placenta
   i. Short umbilical cord
3. If the client is in active labor and bleeding cannot be stopped with bed rest and tocolytic medications, emergency cesarean delivery may be indicated.

**C.** Assessment findings

1. **The client with abruptio placentae may report sudden, intense, localized uterine pain, with or without vaginal bleeding.**
2. Other signs and symptoms of abruptio placentae
   a. Concealed or external dark red bleeding
   b. Uterus firm to boardlike, with severe continuous pain

c. **Uterine outline possibly enlarged or changing shape**

    d. FHR present or absent

**3.** Fetal presenting part may be engaged.

**4.** Severe abruptio placentae may produce such complications as:

    a. Hemorrhage and shock

    b. Renal failure

    c. Disseminated intravascular coagulation

    d. Maternal and fetal death

**D. Nursing diagnoses**

  **1.** Fear

  **2.** Risk for Fluid Volume Deficit

  **3.** Knowledge Deficit

  **4.** Pain

**E. Planning and implementation**

  **1.** Continuously evaluate maternal and fetal physiologic status, particularly:

    a. Vital signs

    b. Bleeding

    c. Electronic fetal and maternal monitoring tracings

    d. Signs of shock—rapid pulse, pallor, cold and moist skin, decrease in blood pressure

    e. Decreasing urine output

   **2. Never perform a vaginal or rectal examination or take any action that would stimulate uterine activity.**

  **3.** Provide emotional support, and teach about the condition.

  **4.** Assess the need for immediate delivery.

**F. Evaluation**

  **1.** The client remains free from complications.

  **2.** Pregnancy progresses to delivery without further incident.

## X. PIH

**A. Description**

   **1. PIH is a hypertensive disorder of pregnancy developing after 20 weeks' gestation and characterized by edema, hypertension, and proteinuria.**

  **2.** PIH can take two forms: preeclampsia and eclampsia.

**B. Etiology and pathophysiology**

  **1.** The cause of PIH is unknown.

  **2.** Possible contributing factors

    a. Poor prenatal care, particularly inadequate nutrition

    b. Primigravid status

    c. Multiple pregnancy

    d. Preexisting maternal diabetes mellitus or hypertension

    e. Age younger than 18 or older than 35 years

    f. Inadequate prenatal care
    g. Race (other than white)
    h. Hydatidiform mole
    i. Low socioeconomic status

 **1.** **Warning signs of worsening preeclampsia**
    a. **Rapid rise in blood pressure**
    b. **Rapid weight gain**
    c. **Generalized edema**
    d. **Increased proteinuria**
    e. **Epigastric pain, marked hyperreflexia, or severe headache, all of which usually precede convulsions in eclampsia**
    f. **Visual disturbances**
    g. **Oliguria (< 120 mL in 4 hours)**
    h. **Irritability**
    i. **Severe nausea and vomiting**

 **2.** Manifestations of mild preeclampsia
    a. Blood pressure exceeding 160/110 mm Hg; increase above baseline of 30 mm Hg in systolic pressure or 15 mm Hg in diastolic pressure on two readings taken 6 hours apart
    b. Generalized edema in face, hands, and ankles—a classic sign
    c. Weight gain of about 1.5 kg (3.3 lb) per month in second trimester or more than 1.3 to 2.3 kg (3–5 lb) per week in third trimester
    d. Proteinuria 1+ to 2+

 **3.** Preeclampsia marked by:
    a. Blood pressure exceeding 160/110 mm Hg noted on two readings taken 6 hours apart with the client on bed rest
    b. Proteinuria exceeding 5 g/24 hours
    c. Oliguria (less than 400 mL/24 hours)
    d. Headache
    e. Blurred vision, spots before eyes, retinal edema
    f. Pitting edema of legs
    g. Dyspnea
    h. Epigastric pain
    i. Nausea and vomiting
    j. Hyperreflexia
    k. Anxiety, irritability

 **4.** Eclampsia may produce:
    a. Blood pressure exceeding 160/110 mm Hg
    b. Grand mal (known as generalized or tonic-clonic) seizures

    c.   Coma

  **5.**  Abnormal test results (Table 12-1)

**D.**  **Nursing diagnoses**

  **1.**  Anxiety

  **2.**  Risk for Injury

  **3.**  Knowledge Deficit

  **4.**  Pain

**E.**  **Planning and implementation**

  **1.**  Monitor vital signs and FHR.

  **2.**  Minimize external stimuli; promote rest and relaxation.

  **3.**  Measure and record urine output, protein level, and specific gravity.

  **4.**  Assess for edema of face, arms, hands, legs, ankles, and feet. Also assess for pulmonary edema.

  **5.**  Weigh client daily.

  **6.**  Assess deep tendon reflexes every 4 hours.

  **7.**  Assess for placental separation, headache and visual disturbance, epigastric pain, and altered level of consciousness.

  **8.**  Provide treatment as prescribed, which may include:

    a.  For mild preeclampsia: bed rest in left lateral recumbent position, balanced diet with moderate to high protein and low to moderate sodium, magnesium sulfate

    b.  For severe preeclampsia: complete bed rest, balanced

TABLE 12-1.
Significant Laboratory Findings in PIH

| TEST | FINDINGS |
| --- | --- |
| **Blood** | |
| Hematocrit | >40% |
| **Renal Function** | |
| Serum uric acid | ≥5.5 mg/dL<br>>6.0 mg/dL (severe pregnancy-induced hypertension [PIH]) |
| Creatinine | ≥1.0 mg/dL<br>2.0–3.0 mg/dL (severe PIH) |
| Creatinine clearance | <150 mL/min |
| BUN | 8–10 mg/dL<br>10–16 mg/dL (severe PIH) |
| **Coagulation** | |
| Platelets | <100,000 µL (severe PIH) |
| Fibrin degradation products | ≥ 16 ug/mL (severe PIH) |

diet with high protein and low to moderate sodium, sulfate, fluid and electrolyte replacements, and sedative antihypertensives, such as diazepam or phenobarbital, or an anticonvulsant such as phenytoin.

   c.   For eclampsia: magnesium sulfate intravenously

9. Institute seizure precautions. Seizures may occur up to 72 hours after delivery.

10. Offer emotional support.

**F.** **Evaluation**

1. The client remains free of serious complications or exhibits resolution of complications.

2. The client verbalizes understanding of the disorder and treatment measures.

3. Pregnancy progresses to term without major incident.

# XI. Gestational diabetes

**A.** **Description**

1. Abnormal carbohydrate, fat, and protein metabolism first diagnosed during pregnancy, also called class A diabetes

2. Usually requires diet therapy to control carbohydrate, fat, and protein intake; also may require insulin injection (two types: type I, or insulin-dependent diabetes mellitus, and type II, non–insulin-dependent diabetes mellitus)

3. About 15,000 infants born yearly to mothers with diabetes

**B.** **Etiology and pathophysiology**

1. The cause of type I diabetes, characterized by a loss of beta pancreatic cells, is unknown. However, inheritance, autoimmune response, and viruses (eg, coxsackie, mumps, and congenital rubella) may be factors. The condition may have multiple causes. Type I is more like to occur in pregnant women.

2. The cause of type II diabetes also is largely unknown but may be related to genetics or obesity. Although individuals with type II diabetes have a normal number of insulin-producing beta cells, they either fail to release insulin as needed or respond abnormally to insulin at the tissue level.

3. In gestational diabetes mellitus (type III, GDM), insulin antagonism by placental hormones, human placental lactogen, progesterone, cortisol, and prolactin, leads to increased blood glucose levels. The effect of these hormones peaks at about 26 weeks' gestation. This is called the diabetogenic effect of pregnancy.

4. Since 1980, the International Workshop-Conference on Gestational Diabetes and the American Diabetes Association have recommended universal screening for gestational diabetes.

**C. Assessment findings**

1. Client may report increased appetite, thirst, and urine volume with weight loss and decreased muscle strength.
2. Client history may include risk factors for glucose intolerance:
   a. Family history of diabetes (parents and siblings)
   b. Poor obstetric history, including spontaneous abortions, unexplained stillbirth, unexplained hydramnios, premature birth, low birth weight or birth weight exceeding 4,000 g (8 lb, 13 oz), birth of newborn with congenital anomalies, five or more pregnancies, maternal age over 35
   c. Obesity
   d. Recurrent monilial vaginitis
   e. Glycosuria
   f. Possibly stress-related precipitators, such as family problems, socioeconomic status, cultural expectations, religious beliefs, level of education
3. Physical examination should include:
   a. Maternal height, weight, and blood pressure
   b. Determination of FHR
   c. Thyroid palpation (Typically thyroid disorders are associated with diabetes.)
   d. Characteristics of vascular system and circulation (palpation of pulse points, particularly peripheral and pedal pulses)
   e. Routine prenatal laboratory test findings
   f. Client's mastery of diabetic self-care measures, including diabetic diet and self-administration of insulin if appropriate
4. Diagnostic test findings related to GDM
   a. Fasting blood sugar
   b. 50-g glucose screen: Blood glucose level is measured 1 hour after client ingests a 50-g glucose drink; test can be done without regard to time of day or last oral intake. Normal plasma threshold is 135–140 mg/dL.
   c. Three-hour oral glucose tolerance test: This is performed if 50-g glucose screen results are abnormal (Table 12-2).
   d. Glycosylated hemoglobin (HbA 1c) test: This measures glycemic control in the 4 to 8 weeks before test; results reflect enzymatic bonding of glucose to hemoglobin A amino acids. This is a useful indicator of overall blood glucose control.
   e. Lipid profile (high- and low-density lipoprotein cholesterol and triglycerides)
   f. Serum creatinine
   g. Urinalysis

TABLE 12–2.
Normal Glucose Tolerance Test Values

| TEST TIMING | VENOUS PLASMA | WHOLE BLOOD |
|---|---|---|
| Fasting | <105 mg/dL | <90 mg/dL |
| 1h | <190 mg/dL | <170 mg/dL |
| 2h | <165 mg/dL | <145 mg/dL |
| 3h | <145 mg/dL | <125 mg/dL |

    h.   Urine culture
    i.   Thyroid function tests ($T_4$ or TSH)
    j.   Electrocardiogram
    k.   Screens for fetal (and later, neonatal) complications, including:

> ▸ Maternal serum alpha-fetoprotein level to assess risk for neural tube defects in newborn
> ▸ Ultrasonography to detect fetal structural anomalies, macrosomia, and hydramnios
> ▸ Nonstress test (as early as 30 weeks), contraction stress test, and biophysical profile because of risk of unexplained intrauterine fetal demise in antepartum period
> ▸ Lung maturity studies (by amniocentesis) to determine lecithin-sphingomyelin (L/S) ratio and to detect phosphatidylglycerol (PG); the adequacy of L/S and PG, predictor of the newborn's ability to avoid respiratory distress (see "Newborn of a diabetic mother" in Chap. 15)

**D.**  **Nursing diagnoses**
    **1.**  Altered Nutrition: More than body requirements
    **2.**  Altered Nutrition: Less than body requirements
    **3.**  Knowledge Deficit
    **4.**  Risk for Infection
    **5.**  Altered Tissue Perfusion: Uteroplacental
    **6.**  Anxiety
    **7.**  Fear
    **8.**  Powerlessness
    **9.**  Ineffective Individual Coping
    **10.**  Noncompliance
    **11.**  Body Image Disturbance
    **12.**  Anticipatory Grieving

**E.**  **Planning and implementation**
    **1.**  Assess client's feelings about herself and the pregnancy.
    **2.**  Review pertinent health history and history of current pregnancy.

3. Assess client's understanding of GDM and its implications for daily life.

4. As needed, explain the effects of gestational diabetes on the mother and fetus.

5. Point out the need for frequent laboratory testing and follow-up for mother and fetus, for example, to prevent infection and assess other potential complications.

6. Establish initial data base, and maintain serial documentation of test results.

7. Provide pertinent client instruction:

   a. Discuss and demonstrate insulin self-injection.

   b. Demonstrate how to self-monitor blood glucose level. Explain that blood is generally tested daily before meals and at bedtime.

   c. Point out the importance of keeping daily records of blood glucose values, insulin dose, dietary intake, periods of exercise, periods of hypoglycemia, kind and amount of treatment, and daily urine test results.

   d. Discuss potential complications, such as diabetic ketoacidosis, a multisystem disorder resulting from hyperglycemia in which plasma glucose levels exceed 350 mg/dL (Table 12-3), or hypoglycemia, a disorder caused by too much insulin, insufficient food, excess exercise, diarrhea, or vomiting. Identify signs and symptoms of hypoglygcemia including:

      ▶ Hunger
      ▶ Nervousness
      ▶ Weakness, fatigue, dizziness, headache, blurred vision
      ▶ Sweating, pallor, shallow respirations but normal pulse rate
      ▶ Urine negative for glucose and acetone
      ▶ Blood glucose level below 60 mg/dL

   e. Discuss management of hypoglycemia by administering 12 fluid oz of orange juice (or 20 g carbohydrate) and waiting 20 minutes before repeating procedure. Report episode to health care provider as soon as possible.

TABLE 12–3.
Laboratory Values in Diabetic Ketoacidosis (DKA)

| DEGREE OF DKA | TOTAL $CO_2$ | PH |
|---|---|---|
| Mild | 21–28 mEq/L | ≥7.30 |
| Moderate | 11–20 mEq/L | 7.10–7.30 |
| Severe | ≤ 10 mEq/L | <7.10 |

      f.   Explain the need to test urine for ketones, which are harmful to the fetus.

  **8.**  Arrange for client to consult with dietitian to discuss prescribed diabetic diet and to ensure adequate caloric intake (Table 12-4).

  **9.**  Explore fears and misconceptions, and intervene appropriately to allay anxiety regarding diabetes and childbirth.

  **10.**  Provide opportunities for anticipatory grieving as needed by client and family.

  **11.**  Prepare the client for intensive frequent intrapartum assessment, which may include:

      a.   Fetal monitoring

      b.   Intravenous infusion of glucose, insulin, and oxytocin

      c.   Evaluation for diabetic ketoacidosis (signs and symptoms include altered level of consciousness, labored breath sounds, fruity breath odor, and ketonuria)

      d.   Intravenous fluid and electrolyte replacement therapy

      e.   Invasive maternal cardiac monitoring

  **12.**  Identify and make referral to support groups and resources available to the client and family.

  **13.**  Explain the need for continued evaluation during the postpartum period until blood glucose levels are within normal limits.

**F.**  **Evaluation**

  **1.**  Antepartum—client

      a.   Achieves and maintains blood glucose levels within normal limits

      b.   Demonstrates appropriate blood glucose self-monitoring skills

      c.   Verbalizes understanding of diabetic diet

      d.   Demonstrates appropriate insulin administration

      e.   Correctly identifies measures to prevent, recognize, or treat hypoglycemia and diabetic ketoacidosis

TABLE 12–4.
**Generally Recommended Caloric Intake for Pregnant Diabetic Women**

| CATEGORY | KCAL/LB PER DAY | TOTAL GAIN |
|---|---|---|
| Adult | 16.4 | 24–30 lb |
| Adolescent | 20.5 | 30 lb |
| Underweight | 22.7 | 30 lb |
| Obese | 13.6 | 20 lb |

       f.   Sustains appropriate weight gain

       g.   Remains free of infection

2. Antepartum—fetus
   a. Grows appropriately
   b. Evidences no clinical signs of complications
3. Intrapartum—client
   a. Sustains blood glucose level within a range of 60 to 100 mg/dL
   b. Shows no clinical signs or symptoms of hypoglycemia
   c. Maintains fluid and electrolyte balance
   d. Is alert and oriented with normal respiratory function
   e. Remains free of diabetic ketoacidosis
4. The intrapartum fetus has a normal heart rate within the range of 120 to 160 beats/min.
5. Postpartum—client
   a. Achieves and maintains euglycemia (blood glucose levels within normal limits)
   b. Remains free of complications
   c. Experiences pregnancy and birth in a positive way
   d. Demonstrates positive health maintenance behaviors
6. The postpartum newborn experiences no complications following birth.

## XII. Hemolytic disease of the fetus and newborn

**A. Description: an immune reaction by the mother's blood against the blood group factor on the fetus' red blood cells**

**B. Etiology and pathophysiology**

1. This disorder occurs when the fetus inherits a blood group antigen from the father that the mother does not possess. The mother's body forms an antibody against that particular blood group antigen, and hemolysis begins.
2. Hemolytic disease may result from ABO or Rh incompatibility. ABO incompatibility occurs in about 20% of pregnancies, Rh in about 1.5%.
3. When RhoGAM (Rh immune globulin) became available in the 1960s to treat isoimmunization in Rh-negative women, the incidence of hemolytic disease in the fetus and newborn dropped.

**C. Assessment findings**

1. The hemolytic response in ABO incompatibility is usually mild, and phototherapy usually can resolve the resulting newborn jaundice.
2. In the Rh-negative mother, Rh incompatibility leads to varying degrees of anemia and jaundice (erythroblastosis fetalis) if the fetus is Rh positive.

**D.** **Nursing diagnoses**
1. Anxiety
2. Knowledge Deficit
3. Fear

**E.** **Planning and Implementation**
1. Provide appropriate and accurate information relative to the treatment and care anticipated.

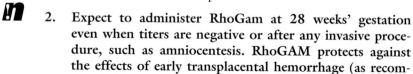 2. **Expect to administer RhoGam at 28 weeks' gestation even when titers are negative or after any invasive procedure, such as amniocentesis. RhoGAM protects against the effects of early transplacental hemorrhage (as recommended by the American College of Gynecologists).**

3. Ensure that the mother is cross-matched with RhoGam; coordination with the laboratory for the injection setup is necessary.

4. Focus management of the immunized Rh-negative mother on close monitoring of fetal well-being, as reflected by Rh titers, amniocentesis results, and sonography.

5. **When the Rh-negative mother is in labor, cross-match for RhoGAM, which is to be given within 72 hours of delivery.**

6. If the mother becomes sensitized and there is evidence of erythroblastosis, notify the perinatal team of the possibility for delivery of a compromised newborn.

**F.** **Evaluation**
1. The client responds to treatment; antibody titers remain within normal limits.
2. The client continues follow-up appointments to assess progress of pregnancy and effectiveness of treatment.

## Bibliography

Bobak, I. M., & Jensen, M. D. (1993). *Maternity and gynecologic care: The nurse and the family* (5th ed.). St. Louis: C.V. Mosby.

Mandeville, L. K., & Troiano, N. H. (1992). *NAACOG: High-risk intrapartum nursing.* Philadelphia: J.B. Lippincott.

May, K. A., & Mahlmeister, L. R. (1994). *Maternal and neonatal nursing: Family-centered care* (3rd ed.). Philadelphia: J.B. Lippincott.

McElmurry, B. J., & Parker, R. S. (Ed.) (1993). *Annual review of women's health.* New York: National League for Nursing.

Olds, S. B., London, M. L., & Ladewig, P. W. (1992). *Maternal-newborn nursing: A family centered approach* (4th ed.). Menlo Park, CA: Addison-Wesley.

Reeder, S. J., Martin, L. L., & Koniak, D. (1992). *Maternity nursing: Family newborn, and women's health care* (17th ed.). Philadelphia: J.B. Lippincott.

## STUDY QUESTIONS

1. Select from the following the best description of hyperemesis gravidarum:
   a. Severe anemia leading to electrolyte, metabolic, and nutritional imbalances in the absence of other medical problems
   b. Severe nausea and vomiting leading to electrolyte, metabolic, and nutritional imbalances in the absence of other medical problems
   c. Loss of appetite and continuous vomiting that commonly results in dehydration and ultimately decreases the mother's amount of circulating nutrients
   d. Severe nausea and diarrhea that can cause gastrointestinal irritation and possibly internal bleeding

2. Which of the following is the best description of anemia?
   a. Hemoglobin value of 12 g or less during the first and second trimesters
   b. Hemoglobin value of 6 g or less during the first and second trimesters
   c. Hemoglobin value of 8 g or less during the third trimester
   d. Hemoglobin value of 10 g or less during the second and third trimesters

3. Which of the following is a classic sign of PIH?
   a. Edema of the feet and ankles
   b. Edema of the hands and face
   c. Weight gain of 1 lb/week
   d. Early morning headache

4. Identify the best description of hemolytic disease of the fetus and newborn.
   a. An immune reaction of the fetus' blood against the blood group factor on the mother's red blood cells
   b. An immune reaction by the mother's blood against the blood group factor on the fetus' red blood cells

   c. Rh incompatibility disease that results in a hemoglobin value of 10 g or less in the fetus or newborn
   d. Rh disease that results in sickle cell disease in the fetus or newborn

5. Several classifications are used to describe spontaneous abortions. In which type would the findings include dark brown vaginal discharge and a negative pregnancy test?
   a. Threatened
   b. Imminent
   c. Missed
   d. Incomplete

6. From the following, select the predisposing factors that could cause placenta previa:
   a. Multiple gestation
   b. Uterine anomalies
   c. Abdominal trauma
   d. Renal or vascular disease

7. The signs and symptoms of abruptio placentae include which of the following?
   a. Bright red, painless vaginal bleeding
   b. Concealed or external dark red bleeding
   c. Palpable fetal outline
   d. Soft and nontender abdomen

8. Premature separation of a normally implanted placenta during the second half of pregnancy, usually with severe hemorrhage, describes which of the following?
   a. Placenta previa
   b. Ectopic pregnancy
   c. Incompetent cervix
   d. Abruptio placentae

9. Which of the following best describes gestational trophoblastic disease?
   a. It is a hypertensive disorder of pregnancy that develops after 20 weeks' gestation and is characterized by edema, hypertension, and proteinuria.
   b. It is the implantation of products of conception in a site other than the

endometrium (ie, ovary, cervix or peritoneal cavity).

c. It is an alteration of early fetal growth, causing fetal death and rapid proliferation of abnormal cells.

d. It is an alteration of early embryonic growth, causing placental disruption, rapid proliferation of abnormal

cells, and destruction of the embryo.

10. The ingestion of DES by the woman's mother may be one of the causes for which of the following?
   a. Placenta previa
   b. Incompetent cervix
   c. Preeclampsia
   d. Severe eclampsia

For additional questions, see
*Lippincott's Self-Study Series* Software
Available at your bookstore

# ANSWER KEY

**1.** *Correct response: b*
The description of hyperemesis gravidarum includes severe nausea and vomiting, leading to electrolyte, metabolic, and nutritional imbalances in the absence of other medical problems.
**a, c, and d.** These are incorrect answers.
*Comprehension/Safe Care/Assessment*

**2.** *Correct response: d*
The description of anemia is a hemoglobin value of 10 g or less during the second and third trimesters.
**a.** A hemoglobin value of 12 is sufficient, but it must stay at that level through all three trimesters.
**b and c.** These are insufficient hemoglobin levels regardless of the trimester.
*Knowledge/Safe Care/Implementation*

**3.** *Correct response: b*
Edema of the hands and face is a classic sign of PIH
**a.** Many healthy pregnant women experience foot and ankle edema.
**c.** Weight gain of 2 lb or more per week indicates a problem.
**d.** Early morning headache is not a classic sign of PIH.
*Knowledge/Safe Care/Assessment*

**4.** *Correct response: b*
Hemolytic disease of the fetus and newborn is caused by an immune reaction by the mother's blood against the blood group factor on the fetus' red blood cells.
**a, c, and d.** All are incorrect.
*Knowledge/Safe Care/Assessment*

**5.** *Correct response: c*
In a missed abortion, there is early fetal intrauterine death, and products of conception are not expelled. The cervix remains closed; there may be a dark brown vaginal discharge, negative pregnancy test, and cessation of uterine growth and breast tenderness.
**a, b, and d.** These are all types of spontaneous abortions, but none is characterized by dark brown vaginal discharge and negative pregnancy test results.
*Comprehension/Safe Care/Assessment*

**6.** *Correct response: a*
One of the predisposing factors that may cause placenta previa is multiple gestation.
**b, c, and d.** These are predisposing factors that may cause abruptio placentae.
*Comprehension/ Physiologic/Assessment*

**7.** *Correct response: b*
One of the signs and symptoms of abruptio placentae is concealed or dark red bleeding.
**a, c, and d.** These are all signs and symptoms related to placenta previa.
*Knowledge/Safe Care/Assessment*

**8.** *Correct response: d*
The description of abruptio placentae is premature separation of a normally implanted placenta during the second half of pregnancy, often with severe hemorrhage.
**a, b, and c.** These complications may cause vaginal bleeding, with minor pain and concern.
*Knowledge/Safe Care/Assessment*

**9.** *Correct response: d*
Gestational trophoblastic disease (hydatidiform mole) is an alteration of early embryonic growth, causing placental disruption, rapid proliferation of abnormal cells, and destruction of the embryo.
**a.** This describes PIH.
**b.** This describes ectopic pregnancy.
**c.** This an incorrect answer.
*Knowledge/Safe Care/Assessment*

**10.** *Correct response: b*

One of the causes of incompetent cervix may be that the woman's mother took DES during pregnancy.

**a, c, and d.** All are incorrect answers.

*Knowledge/Safe Care/Assessment*

# Intrapartum Complications

## I. Overview

### A. Essential concepts

1. Problems that can be anticipated because of maternal or fetal conditions or that can be stabilized and corrected without emergency intervention are increasingly managed in facilities designed to accommodate high-risk maternal and fetal clients.

2. When the expectant mother is the best "incubator" for the high-risk newborn, she may be transported to a tertiary care facility.

3. **Because intrapartum emergencies commonly develop rapidly, on-the-spot nursing assessment and intervention are crucial.**

4. Principles of nursing care during normal labor (see Chap. 9) apply to complicated labor as well.

### B. General nursing management of at-risk intrapartum clients

1. Assessment
   a. Review maternal health history.
   b. Review history of previous pregnancies.
   c. Identify predisposing factors for intrapartum complications.
   d. Continuously assess maternal physiologic status to detect early maternal or fetal changes requiring early intervention.
   e. Assess the family's responses to labor and a potential crisis situation.
   f. **Accurately document the assessed problem and subsequent nursing interventions and their effectiveness.**

2. Nursing diagnoses: In addition to complication-specific diagnoses, the following nursing diagnoses are common to care of the at-risk intrapartum client:
   a. Anxiety
   b. Decreased Cardiac Output
   c. Ineffective Compromised Family Coping
   d. Anticipatory Grieving
   e. Risk for Injury
   f. Knowledge Deficit
   g. Fear
   h. Pain
   i. Self Esteem Disturbance
   j. Spiritual Distress
   k. Altered Tissue Perfusion
   l. Altered Urinary Elimination

3.  Planning and implementation
    a.  Assess and support maternal and fetal physiologic status.
    b.  Provide anticipatory guidance for the client and her partner.
    c.  Coordinate client care. (Typically, clients with intra-partum complications require intravenous fluids and various procedures and treatments, such as electronic monitoring, central venous lines, medications, and re-tention catheters.)

 d.  **Expect the unexpected, and be prepared to provide critical care nursing if needed.**
4.  Evaluation
    a.  The client and fetus maintain normal physiologic status; any deviations that arise are identified and corrected early.
    b.  The client and partner express understanding of proce-dures to be performed.
    c.  The couple demonstrates decreased fear and anxiety, greater comfort, and increased use of coping tech-niques.

## II. Induction of labor
### A. Overview
1.  The deliberate initiation of labor before spontaneous contrac-tions begin may be either mechanical (amniotomy or rupture of amniotic membranes), physiologic (ambulation, nipple stimulation), or chemical (prostaglandins and oxytocin).
2.  Artificial rupture of membranes (AROM) may be adequate stimulation to initiate contractions, or AROM may be done after oxytocin administration establishes effective contrac-tions.

 3.  **AROM is initiated when the cervix is soft, partially ef-faced, and slightly dilated, preferably when the fetal pre-senting part is engaged.**

 4.  **Oxytocin-induced labor must be done with careful, on-going monitoring; oxytocin is a powerful drug. Hy-perstimulation of the uterus may result in tetanic con-tractions prolonged to more than 90 seconds, which could cause such complications as fetal distress due to im-paired uteroplacental perfusion, abruptio placentae, am-niotic fluid embolism, laceration of the cervix and uterine rupture, and neonatal trauma.**
### B. Nursing implications: AROM
1.  Explain the procedure, and inform the client that labor usu-

ally follows within 6 to 8 hours of AROM. Prepare the client to expect intense contractions and leakage of fluid.

2. Monitor fetal heart tones immediately before, during, and after the procedure.

***n*** 3. **Observe and record color, amount, and odor of fluid; time of procedure; cervical status; and maternal temperature.**

4. Take and record the client's temperature every 2 hours to assess for infection.

C. **Nursing management: Oxytocin-induced labor**

1. Review the hospital's policy relative to the amount, rate, and interval for increasing oxytocin.

2. Use infusion pump for precise regulation of the medication.

3. Observe for signs of hypertonicity, such as contractions exceeding 75 mm Hg, exceeding 90 seconds, or closer than 2 minutes. Be prepared to discontinue the oxytocin immediately.

4. Initiate continuous internal or external fetal monitoring, and evaluate for normal range of 120 to 160 beats/min. If there is loss of variability, late decelerations, or persistent bradycardia (fewer than 120 beats/min), discontinue oxytocin infusion, administer $O_2$, notify physician, reposition client to left or right side, and perform a vaginal examination; fetal distress may result from rapid labor progress, descent of fetus, or cord prolapse.

***n*** 5. **Assess and record vital signs and fetal heart rate (FHR) every 15 to 30 minutes; assess for signs of impending delivery.**

**III. Cesarean delivery**

A. Overview

1. In this surgical procedure, the newborn is delivered through an incision made through the maternal abdomen.

2. The surgery may be planned (elective) or arise from an unanticipated problem (emergency).

3. Types of cesarean delivery

a. Classic: A vertical midline skin incision is made in the skin and the body of the uterus, permitting easier access to the fetus; this is indicated in emergency situations, when there are abdominal adhesions from previous surgeries, or when the fetus is in a transverse lie. Blood loss is increased because large blood vessels of the myometrium are involved. Because the uterine musculature is weakened, there is greater possibility of rupture of the uterine scar in subsequent pregnancies.

b. Low segment: In this, the most common type, the incision is low ("bikini" or Pfannenstiel's incision), and the uterine incision is horizontal in the lower uterine segment. Blood loss is minimal, fewer postdelivery complications occur, and the incision is easy to repair, with less chance of rupture of uterine scar during future deliveries. The procedure takes longer to perform than the classic incision; it is therefore not useful in emergencies.

4. In subsequent pregnancies and delivery, a trial of labor and vaginal birth is increasingly regarded as safe and appropriate.

5. Elective, repeat cesarean may be performed in the absence of a specific indication for operative delivery when either the physician or the client is unwilling to attempt vaginal delivery.

6. Anesthesia may be general, spinal, or epidural; preoperative and postoperative care will vary accordingly.

**B. Assessment**

1. Obtain a complete obstetric history.
2. Assess condition and signs of labor.
3. Determine frequency, duration, and intensity of contractions.
4. Determine condition of fetus through fetal heart tones, fetal monitoring strips, fetal scalp blood sample, fetal activity changes, and presence of meconium in amniotic fluid.
5. Observe the client and family for emotional response and ability to cope with discomfort and pain.

**C. Nursing diagnoses**

1. Anxiety
2. Body Image Disturbance
3. Ineffective Individual Coping
4. Fear
5. Risk for Fluid Volume Deficit
6. Risk for Injury
7. Knowledge Deficit
8. Pain
9. Altered Urinary Elimination

**D. Planning and implementation**

1. **Modify preoperative teaching to meet the needs of planned versus emergency cesarean birth; depth and breadth of instruction will depend on the circumstances and time available.**

2. Facilitate a family-centered cesarean birth by including, when possible, such activities as:

   a. Preparing the partner for participation in the delivery

    b.    Reuniting the family as soon as possible following delivery

    c.    Providing for family time alone in the critical first hours after the mother and newborn are stabilized

    d.    Including the father and siblings (as possible) when demonstrating care of the newborn

3.    Prepare the woman for cesarean delivery in the same way whether the surgery is elective or emergency. Depending on hospital policy:

    a.    Shave or clip pubic hair.

    b.    Insert a retention catheter to empty the bladder continuously.

    c.    As prescribed, insert intravenous lines, collect specimens for laboratory analysis, and administer preoperative medications.

    d.    Also as prescribed, provide an antacid (to prevent vomiting and possible aspiration of gastric secretions) and prophylactic antibiotics (to prevent endometritis).

    e.    Assist the client to remove jewelry, dentures, and nail polish as appropriate.

4.    As needed, reinforce the obstetrician's explanation of the surgery, the expected outcome, and the anesthesiologist's explanation of the kind of anesthetics to be used (depending on the client's cardiopulmonary status).

5.    Make sure the client's signed informed consent is on file.

6.    **Continue assessing maternal and fetal vital signs in accordance with hospital policy until the client is transported to the operating room.**

7.    Notify other health care team members of the pending delivery.

8.    Encourage the mother's support person to remain with her as much as possible. In some cases, this person may accompany the client to the surgical suite and stay with her throughout the birth.

9.    If there is time, begin explaining what the client can expect postoperatively. Discuss pain relief, turning, coughing, deep-breathing, and ambulation.

10.    Inform the client that intraoperative and postpartum care will be performed by the surgical and obstetric team and that the newborn will receive care by the pediatrician and a nurse skilled in neonatal care procedures (ie, resuscitation).

11.    Continuously assess maternal physiologic status to detect early maternal or fetal changes requiring rapid intervention.

12.    Anticipate parental feelings of "failure" related to cesarean rather than "normal" birth. In such a situation, provide time

for them to relive and talk through the experience. Offer reassurance and support.

13. Refer for home care and follow-up visit, as indicated by mother's and newborn's status and length of hospital stay.

14. Assist family in planning for care of mother and newborn at home, taking into consideration the need for increased rest (influenced by type of anesthesia, length of labor, type of abdominal or uterine incision) and the inability to climb stairs and drive a car.

### E. Evaluation

1. The clients progressively recover without complications.

2. The client recovering from cesarean birth responds to analgesics and states that she is comfortable.

3. The client maintains appropriate intake and output and can void when indwelling catheter (Foley) is removed.

4. The client demonstrates beginning of attachment and parenting.

## IV. Preterm labor

### A. Description: labor that begins after 20 weeks' gestation and before 37 weeks' gestation

### B. Etiology and pathophysiology

1. Among the many causes of preterm labor are:
   a. Premature rupture of the membranes (PROM)
   b. Preeclampsia
   c. Hydramnios
   d. Placenta previa
   e. Abruptio placentae
   f. Incompetent cervix
   g. Trauma
   h. Uterine structural anomalies
   i. Multiple gestation
   j. Intrauterine infection
   k. Congenital adrenal hyperplasia
   l. Fetal death

2. Maternal risk factors include age younger than 18 years, history of preterm labors, multiple pregnancy, hydramnios, smoking, poor hygiene, poor nutrition, employment.

### C. Assessment

1. **Manifestations of preterm labor are the same as those of labor at term:**
   a. Rhythmic uterine contractions
   b. Cervical dilation and effacement
   c. Possible rupture of membranes
   d. Expulsion of the cervical mucus plug

        e.    Bloody show

    **2.**    Obstetric history reveals less than 37 weeks' gestation

**D.**   **Nursing diagnoses**

    **1.**    Anxiety

    **2.**    Fear

    **3.**    Risk for Injury

    **4.**    Knowledge Deficit

**E.**   **Planning and implementation**

    **1.**    Obtain a thorough obstetric history.

    **2.**    Assess condition and signs of labor.

    **3.**    Determine frequency, duration, and intensity of uterine contractions.

    **4.**    Determine cervical dilation and effacement.

    **5.**    Assess status of membranes and bloody show.

    **6.**    Evaluate fetus for distress, size, maturity (sonography and lecithin-sphingomyelin ratio).

    **7.**    Using nitrazine paper, test vaginal discharge for amniotic fluid.

    **8.**    If possible, relieve anxiety by providing information of status. Offer additional support.

    **9.**    Provide comfort measures and adequate hydration.

  **10.**    Place client on bed rest in side-lying position.

  **11.**    Administer oxygen, 8 to 12 L/min by mask as required.

  **12.**    Obtain specimens for complete blood count and urinalysis.

  **13.**    Prepare for possible ultrasonography, amniocentesis, tocolytic drug therapy, steroid therapy.

  **14.**    Administer tocolytic (contraction-inhibiting) medications as prescribed.

  **15.**    **Assess for side effects of tocolytic therapy (eg, decreased maternal blood pressure, dyspnea, chest pain, and FHR exceeding 180 beats/min).**

**F.**   **Evaluation**

    **1.**    The client responds to treatment, and preterm labor ceases.

    **2.**    Fetus responds to treatment.

    **3.**    The client verbalizes her fears; cooperates with staff.

    **4.**    The client and family verbalize understanding of medical procedures and expected neonatal outcome.

    **5.**    The client copes with decreased mobility and states the reasons for limiting activity.

**V.**   **PROM**

    **A.**   **Description: rupture of the chorion and amnion 1 hour or more before the onset of labor**

    **B.**   **Etiology and pathophysiology**

        **1.**    The precise cause and specific predisposing factors are unknown.

2. PROM is associated with malpresentation, possible weak areas in the amnion and chorion, subclinical infection, and possibly incompetent cervix.

3. Amniotic fluid leaks from the vagina in the absence of contractions.

4. Risk of ascending intrauterine infection known as chorioamnionitis is increased.

 **5. Basic and effective defense against fetus contracting infection is lost; the leading cause of death associated with PROM is infection.**

6. When the latent period (time between rupture of membranes and onset of labor) is less than 24 hours, the risk of infection is low.

7. Management is affected by the gestational age of the fetus and estimates of viability.

**C. Assessment**

1. PROM is marked by amniotic fluid gushing from the vagina.

 **2. Maternal fever, fetal tachycardia, and malodorous discharge may indicate infection.**

**D. Nursing diagnoses**

1. Anxiety
2. Fear
3. Risk for Infection
4. Risk for Injury
5. Knowledge Deficit

**E. Planning and implementation**

1. Determine maternal and fetal status, including estimated gestational age.

 **2. Make an early and accurate evaluation of membrane status, using sterile speculum examination and nitrazine paper testing; thereafter, keep vaginal examinations to a minimum.**

3. Obtain smear specimens from vagina and rectum as prescribed to test for beta-hemolytic streptococci, an organism that increases the risk to the fetus.

4. If leaking amniotic fluid is suspected, assess periodically for early signs of infection.

5. Inform the client, if the fetus is at term, that the chances of spontaneous labor beginning are excellent; encourage the client and partner to prepare themselves for labor and birth.

6. If labor does not begin or the fetus is judged to be preterm or at risk for infection, explain treatments that are likely to be needed.

    7. Maintain client on bed rest if fetal head is not engaged. This may prevent cord prolapse if additional rupture and loss of fluid occur.

  **F.** **Evaluation**

    1. The client and family verbalize understanding of the situation and cooperate with care.

    2. The client and fetus experience no further complications, and delivery progresses.

**VI.** **Dystocia**

  **A.** **Description: difficult, painful, prolonged labor due to mechanical factors**

  **B.** **Etiology and pathophysiology**

    1. Fetal factors (passenger): unusually large fetus, fetal anomaly, malpresentation, malposition

    2. Uterine factors (powers): hypotonic labor, hypertonic labor, precipitous labor, prolonged labor

    3. Pelvic factors (passage): inlet contracture, midpelvis contracture, outlet contracture

    4. "Psyche" factors: maternal anxiety and fear, lack of preparation

  **C.** **Assessment**

    1. Dystocia is marked by decreased strength of uterine contractions and decreased uterine tone after the onset of true labor.

    **2.** **Contractions may become farther apart and irregular.**

  **D.** **Nursing diagnoses**

    1. Anxiety

    2. Fear

    3. Risk for Fluid Volume Deficit

    4. Risk for Infection

    5. Risk for Injury

    6. Knowledge Deficit

    7. Pain

  **E.** **Planning and implementation**

    1. Monitor uterine contractions for dysfunctional patterns; use palpation and an electronic monitor.

    2. Assess condition of fetus by monitoring FHR, fetal activity, and color of amniotic fluid.

    3. Check client's level of fatigue and ability to cope with pain.

    4. Assess maternal vital signs: temperature, pulse, respiratory rates, and blood pressure.

    5. Check maternal urine for acetone (an indication of dehydration and exhaustion).

6.  Offer emotional support by explaining progress and proce-
    dures and giving encouragement and appropriate reassurance.
7.  Promote relaxation through bathing and keeping the client
    and bed clean, back rubs, and frequent position changes
    (side-lying); encourage walking if indicated; keep the envi-
    ronment quiet.
8.  Coach the client in breathing and relaxation techniques.
9.  Assess urinary bladder; catheterize as needed.

**F.** **Evaluation**

1.  The client avoids exhaustion.
2.  The client achieves as much comfort as possible.
3.  The client avoids panic and discouragement.
4.  The client avoids bladder distention.
5.  The client retains normal fluid volume.
6.  The client is free of infection.

## VII. Uterine rupture

**A.** **Description:** abrupt tearing of the uterus, either complete (rupture extends through entire uterine wall and uterine contents
spill into the abdominal cavity) or incomplete (rupture extends
through the endometrium and myometrium, but the peritoneum surrounding the uterus remains intact)

**B.** **Etiology and pathophysiology**

1.  The most common predisposing factor is a preexisting scar
    that results in a weakened or defective myometrium that does
    not stretch; this is most frequently indicated in spontaneous
    uterine rupture.
2.  Traumatic uterine rupture may be caused by injury from ob-
    stetric instruments, such as uterine sound or curette used in
    abortion. Rupture also may result from obstetric intervention,
    such as excessive fundal pressure, forceps delivery, violent
    bearing down, tumultuous labor, and fetal shoulder dystocia.

3.  **Spontaneous uterine rupture is most likely to occur after
    previous uterine surgery, grand multiparity combined
    with the use of oxytocic agents, cephalopelvic dispropor-
    tion, malpresentation, or hydrocephalus.**
4.  More severe ruptures pose the risk of irreversible maternal hy-
    povolemic shock or subsequent peritonitis, consequent fetal
    anoxia, and fetal or neonatal death.
5.  Small tears may be asymptomatic and may heal sponta-
    neously, remaining undetected until the stress and strain of a
    subsequent labor.
6.  If the client has signs of possible uterine rupture, vaginal de-
    livery is generally not attempted.

7. If symptoms are not severe, an emergency cesarean delivery may be attempted and the uterine tear repaired.

8. If symptoms are severe, emergency laparotomy will be performed to attempt immediate delivery of the fetus and then establish homeostasis.

**C. Assessment**

1. Signs and symptoms vary from mild to severe, depending on the site and extent of the rupture, degree of extrusion of the uterine contents, and intraperitoneal evidence or absence of spilled amniotic fluid and blood.

2. Common findings
   a. Abdominal pain
   b. Vaginal bleeding
   c. Lack of progress in labor

 3. **Be alert for maternal signs of hypovolemic shock, an indication of complete uterine rupture.**

**D. Nursing diagnoses**

1. Anxiety
2. Fear
3. Fluid Volume Deficit
4. Risk for Injury
5. Knowledge Deficit
6. Pain

**E. Planning and implementation**

1. In the presence of predisposing factors, monitor maternal labor pattern closely for hypertonicity or signs of weakening uterine muscle.

2. Recognize signs of impending rupture, and immediately notify the physician and call for assistance.

 3. **Take these steps in order to prevent or limit hypovolemic shock:**

   ▸ Oxygenate (8–10 L/min using closed mask)
   ▸ Restore circulating volume (one or more IV lines)
   ▸ Drug therapy (be prepared to give digoxin or a similar drug, and have emergency drugs readily available)
   ▸ Evaluate (cause, response to therapy, fetal condition)
   ▸ Remedy the problem (prepare client for surgery; administer antibiotics)

4. Implement the following preparations for surgery:
   a. Monitor maternal blood pressure, pulse, and respirations; also monitor fetal heart tones.
   b. If the client has a central venous pressure catheter in

place, monitor pressure to evaluate blood loss and effects of fluid and blood replacement.

    c.   Insert a urinary catheter for precise determinations of fluid balance.

    d.   Obtain blood to assess possible acidosis.

    e.   Administer oxygen, and maintain a patent airway.

   5.   Provide support for client's partner and family members once surgery has begun; inform them how they will receive information about the mother and newborn.

**F.**   **Evaluation**

   1.   Signs of uterine rupture are recognized immediately; appropriate and timely interventions follow.

   2.   The client and fetus respond to therapeutic interventions without complications.

## VIII. Uterine inversion

**A.**   **Description: The uterus turns completely or partially inside out; it occurs immediately following delivery of the placenta or in the immediate postpartum period.**

**B.**   **Etiology and pathophysiology**

   1.   Forced inversion is caused by excessive pulling of the cord or vigorous manual expression of the placenta or clots from an atonic uterus.

   2.   Spontaneous inversion is due to increased abdominal pressure because of bearing down, coughing, or sudden abdominal muscle contraction.

   3.   Predisposing factors include straining after delivery of placenta, vigorous kneading of the fundus to expel the placenta, manual separation and extraction of the placenta, rapid delivery with multiple gestation, or rapid release of excessive amniotic fluid.

   4.   **Immediate manual replacement of the uterus at the time of inversion will prevent cervical entrapment of the uterus; if reinversion is not performed immediately, rapid and extreme blood loss may occur, resulting in hypovolemic shock.**

**C.**   **Assessment**

   1.   **Be alert for complaints from an unanesthetized client of excruciating pelvic pain with a sensation of extreme fullness extending into the vagina. These symptoms indicate uterine inversion.**

   2.   Once inversion occurs, the client may exhibit a dramatic increase in vaginal bleeding, accompanied by increasing pulse rate or other signs of hemorrhage.

**D. Nursing diagnoses**
1. Fear
2. Fluid Volume Deficit
3. Risk for Injury
4. Pain

**E. Planning and implementation**
1. Recognize signs of impending inversion, and immediately notify the physician and call for assistance.

 2. **Take the steps in order to prevent or limit hypovolemic shock (see Section VIII.E.3).**
3. If manual reinversion is not successful, prepare the client and family for possible general anesthesia and surgery.

**F. Evaluation**
1. Signs of uterine inversion are recognized immediately; appropriate and timely interventions follow.
2. The client and newborn respond to therapeutic interventions without complications.

## IX. Cord prolapse

**A.** Description: descent of the umbilical cord into the vagina before the fetal presenting part and compression of the cord between the presenting part and the maternal pelvis, compromising or completely cutting off fetoplacental perfusion

**B. Etiology and pathophysiology**
1. This occurs most frequently with prematurity, unengaged cephalic presentations with ruptured membranes, and shoulder of footling breech presentations.
2. It may follow rupture of amniotic membranes because the fluid rush may carry the cord along toward the birth canal.
3. It occurs in 1 of 200 pregnancies.

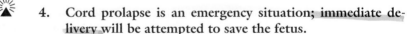 4. **Cord prolapse is an emergency situation; immediate delivery will be attempted to save the fetus.**

**C. Assessment**
1. The prolapsed cord may be visible or palpable.
2. Signs of acute fetal distress may develop as the cord is compressed.

**D. Nursing diagnoses**
1. Anxiety
2. Fear
3. Risk for Injury

**E. Planning and implementation**
1. Assess a laboring client often if the fetus is preterm or small for gestational age, if the fetus has not engaged, or if the client has PROM.

2. Periodically evaluate FHR, especially right after rupture of membranes (spontaneous or surgical) and again in 5 to 10 minutes.

 3. **Lower head of bed and elevate maternal hips on pillow, or place client in knee–chest position to minimize pressure on the cord.**

4. Apply firm upward manual pressure to the presenting part of the fetus with sterile gloved hand to elevate it and relieve pressure from the cord.

5. Assess cord pulsations constantly.

6. Gently wrap gauze soaked in sterile normal saline solution around the prolapsed cord.

7. Notify physician, and prepare for cesarean birth.

8. Provide information and support to woman and family.

   **F.** Evaluation

1. The client and family verbalize understanding of the situation and cooperate with care.

2. The client and fetus experience no further complications, and delivery progresses.

3. The client and family verbalize a decreased level of anxiety.

**X.** **Early postpartum hemorrhage**

   **A.** Description: **blood loss of 500 mL or more during the first 24 hours after delivery** (See Chap. 14 for discussion of hemorrhage that occurs later in the postpartum period.)

   **B.** Etiology and pathophysiology

1. **Postpartum hemorrhage is the leading cause of maternal death worldwide and a common cause of excessive blood loss during early postpartum period.**

2. Approximately 5% of women experience some type of postdelivery hemorrhage.

3. Major causes of postpartum hemorrhage are uterine atony (responsible for at least 80% of all early postpartum hemorrhages); laceration of cervix, vagina, or perineum; and retained placental fragments.

4. Predisposing factors include hypotonic contractions, overdistended uterus, multiparity, large newborn, forceps delivery, and cesarean delivery.

   **C.** Assessment

 1. **Vaginal bleeding is the obvious sign of postpartum hemorrhage; amount and character vary with cause.**

2. Excessive blood loss may produce hypotension, thready pulse, pallor, restlessness, dyspnea, and chills. *Shock*

**D. Nursing diagnoses**
1. Anxiety
2. Body Image Disturbance
3. Decreased Cardiac Output
4. Ineffective Individual and Family Coping
5. Fluid Volume Deficit
6. Impaired Gas Exchange
7. Risk for Injury
8. Knowledge Deficit
9. Pain
10. Powerlessness
11. Altered Tissue Perfusion: Cardiopulmonary

**E. Planning and implementation**
1. Determine presence of uterine atony through frequent periodic assessment of uterine firmness and location and amount of vaginal bleeding immediately after delivery.
2. Measure and record serial maternal vital signs after delivery—every 5 to 15 minutes until stable, increasing or decreasing frequency relative to baseline and amount of bleeding.
3. Massage fundus gently, taking care to support the uterus with the hand just above the symphysis pubis.
4. Administer intravenous oxytocin as prescribed.
5. Keep an accurate pad count (100 mL per saturated pad).
6. Assess condition of skin, urine output, and level of consciousness.
7. Allay anxiety through explanation and reassurance.

**F. Evaluation**
1. The client's condition stabilizes, and she progresses through normal involution.
2. Parent–newborn contact is supported and maintained as the mother's physiologic condition stabilizes.

## Bibliography

Bobak, I. M., & Jensen, M. D. (1993). *Maternity and gynecologic care: The nurse and the family* (5th ed.). St. Louis: C.V. Mosby.

Mandeville, L. K., & Troiano, N. H. (1992). *NAACOG: High-risk intrapartum nursing.* Philadelphia: J.B. Lippincott.

May, K. A., & Mahlmeister, L. R. (1994). *Maternal and neonatal nursing: Family-centered care* (3rd ed.). Philadelphia: J.B. Lippincott.

Olds, S. B., London, M. L., & Ladewig, P. W. (1992). *Maternal-newborn nursing: A family centered approach* (4th ed.). Menlo Park, CA: Addison-Wesley.

Reeder, S. J., Martin, L. L., & Koniak, D. (1992). *Maternity nursing: Family newborn, and women's health care* (17th ed.). Philadelphia: J.B. Lippincott.

# STUDY QUESTIONS

1. Identify what may happen if the uterus becomes overstimulated by oxytocin during the induction of labor.
    a. Hyperstimulation of the uterus may result in weak contractions prolonged to more than 70 seconds.
    **b.** Hyperstimulation of the uterus may result in tetanic contractions prolonged to more than 90 seconds.
    c. The client will report increased pain and have bright red vaginal bleeding.
    d. The client will become more restless and anxious by the overstimulation of the uterus.

2. When preparing a client for cesarean delivery, which of the following key concepts should be considered when implementing nursing care?
    a. Instruct the mother's support person to remain in the family lounge until after the delivery.
    b. Arrange for a staff member of the anesthesia department to explain what to expect postoperatively.
    c. Modify preoperative teaching to meet the needs of either a planned or emergency cesarean birth.
    d. Modify preoperative instruction to meet the needs of the obstetrician and the operating room staff.

3. From the following definitions, select the best description of preterm labor.
    **a.** Labor that begins after 20 weeks' gestation and before 37 weeks' gestation
    b. Labor that begins after 15 weeks' gestation and before 37 weeks' gestation
    c. Labor that begins after 24 weeks' gestation and before 28 weeks' gestation
    d. Labor that begins after 28 weeks' gestation and before 40 weeks' gestation

4. What are the side effects that must be assessed after administering tocolytic medications for a preterm labor client?
    a. Dyspnea, chest pain, decreased urine output, and FHR greater than 180 beats/min
    b. Decreased maternal blood pressure, dyspnea, and FHR less than 180 beats/min
    c. Increased maternal blood pressure, dyspnea, chest pain, and FHR less than 180 beats/min
    d. Decreased maternal blood pressure, dyspnea, chest pain, and FHR greater than 180 beats/min

5. When PROM occurs, which of the following statements would be of immediate importance to the nurse?
    a. The chorion and amnion rupture 4 hours before the onset of labor.
    **b.** PROM removes the fetus' most effective defense against infection.
    c. Nursing care is based on fetal viability and gestational age.
    d. PROM is associated with malpresentation and possibly incompetent cervix.

6. Which of the following is the best description of dystocia?
    a. Difficult, painful, prolonged labor due to nutritional factors
    **b.** Difficult, painful, prolonged labor due to mechanical factors
    c. Difficult, painful, prolonged labor due to environmental factors
    d. Difficult, painful, prolonged labor due to medical factors

7. When uterine rupture occurs, which would be the priority goal of planning and implementing nursing care?
    **a.** Take immediate steps to prevent or limit hypovolemic shock.
    b. Take immediate steps to prevent or limit hypervolemic shock.
    c. Place client on bed rest; monitor maternal vital signs and FHR.
    d. Place client on bed rest, start IV, monitor FHR, and report findings.

**8.** Which of the following may occur in uterine inversion?
   **a.** Along with vaginal hemorrhage, a large mass of tissue appears within the vagina.
   **b.** There will be hemorrhage from the vagina, and the mother will exhibit signs and symptoms of hypervolemic shock.
   **c.** Vaginal bleeding increases dramatically, and the client exhibits signs and symptoms of hypovolemic shock.
   **d.** There is a significant increase in vaginal bleeding. The client complains of pain and becomes cyanotic.

**9.** What is the primary nursing action when the umbilical cord is prolapsed?
   **a.** Place the client on bed rest, and begin monitoring maternal vital signs and FHR.
   **b.** Place the client on bed rest, lower the head of the bed, and elevate the maternal hips on a pillow.
   **c.** Notify the physician, prepare the client for surgery, and monitor the FHR.
   **d.** Place the client on bed rest, and apply sterile warm saline dressing to the exposed cord.

For additional questions, see
*Lippincott's Self-Study Series* Software
Available at your bookstore

# ANSWER KEY

1. **Correct response: b**
   Hyperstimulation of the uterus may result in tetanic contractions prolonged to more than 90 seconds, which could cause such complications as fetal distress, abruptio placentae, amniotic fluid embolism, laceration of the cervix, and uterine rupture.
   **a, c, and d.** All are wrong answers.
   *Application/Physiologic/Analysis (Dx)*

2. **Correct response: c**
   Modify the preoperative teaching to meet the needs of either a planned or emergency cesarean birth; the depth and breadth of instruction will depend on circumstances and time available.
   **a.** Allowing the mother's support person to remain with her as much as possible is an important concept, although doing so depends on many variables.
   **b and d.** These are nursing responsibilities. The anesthesia department (although some staff are nurses), the obstetrician, and the operating room support staff should not be responsible for this part of client care.
   *Application/Safe Care/Implementation*

3. **Correct response: a**
   Preterm labor is described as labor that begins after 20 weeks' gestation and before 37 weeks' gestation.
   **b, c, and d.** All are incorrect answers.
   *Knowledge/Comprehension/Safe Care*

4. **Correct response: d**
   Assess for side effects of tocolytic therapy (eg, decreased maternal blood pressure, dyspnea, chest pain, and FHR greater than 180 beats/min).
   **a, b, and c.** All are incorrect answers.
   *Comprehension/Physiologic/Assessment*

5. **Correct response: b**
   PROM can precipitate many potential and actual problems; one of the most serious is the fetus' loss of an effective

defense against infection, This is the most immediate concern.
   **a.** PROM occurs about 1 hour (not 4 hours) before labor begins.
   **c.** Fetal viability and gestational age are less immediate considerations that affect the plan of care.
   **d.** Malpresentation and an incompetent cervix may be causes of PROM.
   *Application/Safe Care/Implementation*

6. **Correct response: b**
   Dystocia is difficult, painful, prolonged labor due to mechanical factors.
   **a, c, and d.** These may contribute to the mechanical factors that cause dystocia.
   *Knowledge/NA/NA*

7. **Correct response: a**
   Take immediate steps to prevent or limit hypovolemic shock. These should include giving oxygen, replacing lost fluids, providing drug therapy as needed, evaluating fetal responses, and preparing for surgery.
   **b.** This is incorrect.
   **c and d.** These are aspects of care that help prevent hypovolemic shock.
   *Application/Physiologic/Implementation*

8. **Correct response: c**
   Once inversion occurs, the client may exhibit a dramatic increase in vaginal bleeding, accompanied by increasing pulse rate or other signs of hemorrhage.
   **a, b, and d.** These are incorrect answers. The client does not become hypervolemic and rarely will the inverted uterus be seen.
   *Application/Safe Care/Assessment*

9. **Correct response: b**
   The primary intervention involves placing the client on bed rest, lowering the head of the bed, and elevating the maternal hips on a pillow to minimize the pressure on the cord.

a. Bed rest may not be sufficient in this situation.
c. These may be done as part of nursing care, but they do not constitute the primary intervention.

d. The cord may be covered if directed by the physician. However, the primary concern is preventing damage.

*Application/Safe Care/Implementation*

# Postpartum Complications

**14**

## I. Overview

### A. Essential concepts

1. Today, relatively short postpartum hospitalizations (for most clients, 24–72 hours) require the nurse to focus care on assisting parents to care effectively for themselves and their newborns.

2. Preexisting maternal health problems (eg, anemia, pregnancy-induced hypertension, diabetes) contribute to many postpartum complications.

3. Overall nursing objectives for high-risk postpartum clients include:
   a. Prompt diagnosis and treatment of postpartum complications to minimize risk of morbidity, mortality, and dysfunctional effects.
   b. Promote comfort and recovery through physical care measures, nutrition, and pain relief therapies.
   c. Explore the emotional aspects of care of the high-risk newborn and family.
   d. Minimize separation of mother and newborn and assist in developing a bonding relationship through information, support, and encouragement of mother–newborn attachment.
   e. Assist the client and family to deal with anxiety, anger, grief, and fear through self-expression and acceptance.

**B. General nursing management for high-risk postpartum clients**

1. Assess the following:
   a. Vital signs
   b. Patterns of temperature elevation
   c. Condition of perineum and uterus
   d. Character of lochia
   e. Tenderness and pain
   f. Condition of legs
   g. Condition of breasts
   h. Status of bladder and voiding
   i. Rest and sleep
   j. Appetite, nutrition, and hydration
   k. Pain or discomfort
   l. Response to newborn
   m. Response to complication
   n. Response to partner

2. Nursing diagnoses: In addition to complication-specific diagnoses, the following nursing diagnoses are common to at-risk postpartum clients:
   a. Anxiety
   b. Ineffective Individual Coping
   c. Ineffective Family Coping: Compromised
   d. Altered Family Processes
   e. Fear
   f. Knowledge Deficit
   g. Pain
   h. Altered Parenting

3. Planning and implementation
   a. Record and report signs and symptoms of complications.
   b. Administer medications and treatments.
   c. Assess vital signs.
   d. Collect specimens for laboratory testing.
   e. Maintain fluid and hydration status.
   f. Provide physical care.
   g. Enhance fluid and food intake.
   h. Carry out treatment regimen (eg, sitz baths, medications, dressings).
   i. Encourage maximum mother–newborn contact; provide continuous information about the newborn.
   j. Explain and discuss complication, expected course, and treatment.
   k. Involve client's partner in education about complication, newborn, mother's need for emotional support.

4. Evaluation
   a. The mother's vital signs are stable.
   b. The mother voids completely.
   c. The mother remains symptom free.
   d. The mother rests and sleeps well.
   e. The mother takes adequate fluids and food.
   f. The mother reports relief from pain and discomfort.
   g. The mother assumes as much caretaking of newborn as her condition permits.
   h. The mother and newborn begin bonding.
   i. The mother and family understand treatment and expected course of complication.
   j. The mother and family express grief and fear.

## II. Postpartum hemorrhage and subinvolution

### A. Description

1. Postpartum hemorrhage: blood loss of more than 500 mL following birth

 **2. Subinvolution: delayed healing of the placental site**

### B. Etiology and pathophysiology

1. Early postpartum hemorrhage occurs in the first 24 hours after delivery, usually due to uterine atony, lacerations, or retained placental fragments. (See Chap. 13 for information on nursing care related to early postpartum hemorrhage.)

2. Late postpartum hemorrhage occurs after the first 24 hours after delivery and is generally caused by retained placental fragments or bleeding disorders.

3. Subinvolution results from retained placental fragments and

membranes, endometritis, or uterine fibroid tumor; treatment depends on cause.

**C.** **Assessment**

1. Vaginal bleeding is the obvious sign of postpartum hemorrhage; amount and character vary with cause.
2. Signs of impending shock include changes in skin temperature and color and altered level of consciousness.

**D.** **Nursing diagnoses**

1. Anxiety
2. Fear
3. Fluid Volume Deficit
4. Risk for Infection
5. Risk for Injury
6. Knowledge Deficit
7. Pain

**E.** **Planning and implementation**

1. Massage uterus, facilitate voiding, and report blood loss.
2. Prepare for intravenous infusion, oxytocin, and blood transfusions if needed.
3. Administer medications and oxygen as prescribed.
4. Monitor blood pressure and pulse rate every 5 to 15 minutes.
5. Measure and record intake and output.
6. Support and communicate with the client and family members during an emergency situation, thus enhancing cooperation with resuscitative efforts.
7. Demonstrate self-care techniques as appropriate (eg, fundal massage, assessing fundal height and consistency, and inspecting episiotomy and lacerations).
8. Discuss importance of rest and adequate nutrition.

**F.** **Evaluation**

1. The mother's condition stabilizes, and normal involution occurs.
2. The mother can verbalize stages of normal involution and can state danger signs.
3. The mother states how to assess for abnormal bleeding.
4. The mother demonstrates ability to manage self-care.

**III.** **Puerperal infection**

**A.** **Description: infection developing in the birth structures after delivery**

**B.** **Etiology and pathophysiology**

1. Puerperal infection is a major cause of maternal morbidity and mortality. Incidence ranges from 1% to 8% of all deliveries; there is a higher incidence in cesarean deliveries.
2. Major site of postpartum infections is the pelvic cavity; other

common sites include the breasts, urinary tract, and venous system.

 3. **Puerperal morbidity is marked by fever of 38°C (100.4°F) or higher after the first 24 hours postpartum on any 2 of the first 10 postpartum days.**

   4. Causative organisms
      a. Aerobic: beta-hemolytic streptococci, *Escherichia coli, Klebsiella, Proteus mirabilis, Pseudomonas, Staphylococcus aureus,* and *Neisseria*
      b. Anaerobic: *Bacteroides, Peptostreptococcus, Peptococcus,* and *Clostridium perfringens*
   5. Localized infections may affect the vagina, vulva, and perineum.
   6. **Endometritis, localized infection of the uterine lining, occurs 48 to 72 hours after delivery.**
   7. In parametritis (pelvic cellulitis), infection spreads by way of the lymphatics of the connective tissue surrounding the uterus.
   8. Puerperal infection may extend to the peritoneum by way of the lymph nodes and uterine wall.

**C.** **Assessment**
   1. Localized vaginal, vulval, and perineal infections are marked by pain, elevated temperature, edema, redness, firmness and tenderness at site of wound; sensation of heat; burning on urination; and discharge from wound.
   2. Manifestations of endometritis include rise in temperature for several days. In severe endometritis, symptoms include malaise, headache, backache, general discomfort, loss of appetite, large, tender uterus, severe postpartum cramping, brownish-red foul-smelling lochia.
   3. Parametritis (pelvic cellulitis) commonly produces elevated temperature of more than 38.6°C (102°–104°F), chills, abdominal pain, subinvolution of uterus, tachycardia, and lethargy.
   4. Signs and symptoms of peritonitis include high fever, rapid pulse, abdominal pains, nausea, vomiting, and restlessness.

**D.** **Nursing diagnoses**
   1. Risk for Injury
   2. Knowledge Deficit
   3. Pain

**E.** **Planning and implementation**
   1. Inspect perineum twice daily for redness, edema, ecchymosis, and discharge.
   2. Evaluate for abdominal pain, fever, malaise, tachycardia, foul-smelling lochia.

3. Obtain specimens for laboratory analysis; report findings.
4. Offer balanced diet, frequent fluids, and early ambulation.
5. Administer antibiotics or medications as prescribed; document client's response.
6. Describe and demonstrate self-care, stressing careful perineal hygiene and handwashing.

**F.** **Evaluation**
1. The mother remains pain free.
2. The mother performs self-care.
3. The mother verbalizes accurate understanding of her condition.

# IV. Mastitis

**A.** **Description:** inflammation of the breast tissue or abscess formation in glandular tissue

**B.** **Etiology and pathophysiology**
1. Injury to breast is the primary predisposing factor (eg, overdistention, stasis, cracking of nipples).
2. Probable sources of infection
   a. **Epidemic infection: derived from nosocomial source, usually *S. aureus*; localizes in the lactiferous glands and ducts**
   b. Endemic infection: occurs randomly and localizes in the periglandular connective tissue
3. Largely preventable by prophylactic measures, such as good breast hygiene

**C.** **Assessment**
1. Clinical manifestations
   a. Elevated temperature, chills
   b. Increased pulse rate
   c. Engorgement, hardness, and reddening of breasts
   d. Nipple soreness, fissures
   e. Swollen, tender axillary lymph nodes

2. **Because symptoms usually do not occur until the third or fourth postpartum week, teach the client to recognize signs and symptoms of mastitis and to report them to her nurse or physician.**

**D.** **Nursing diagnoses**
1. Anxiety
2. Risk for Injury
3. Knowledge Deficit
4. Pain
5. Altered Parenting

**E.** **Planning and implementation**

1. Observe for elevated temperature, chills, tachycardia, headache, pain and tenderness, firmness, and redness of breast.
2. Prevent infection through meticulous handwashing and prompt attention to blocked milk ducts.
3. Teach mother to breast-feed frequently, adequate breast and nipple care (adequate around-the-clock nonconstrictive support of the breasts, gentleness during care, avoidance of harsh cleansing agents and decrusting the nipple, frequent breast pad changes, intermittent exposure of nipples to the air), and signs and symptoms of infection.
4. Administer antibiotics, and explain importance of following through with prescribed regimen even when symptoms subside.
5. Offer comfort measures, such as small side pillows, icecaps, or heat application over localized abscess.

**F.** **Evaluation**

1. The mother reports decreased pain in breasts and can continue nursing newborn.
2. The mother demonstrates correct breast hygiene and breast-feeding techniques.
3. The mother verbalizes correct understanding of early signs and symptoms of mastitis.
4. If the mother must discontinue breast-feeding, she can accept the adjustment.
5. The mother follows through with antibiotic regimen as prescribed.

**V.** **Thrombophlebitis and thrombosis**

**A.** **Description**

1. Thrombophlebitis is an inflammation of the vascular endothelium with clot formation on the vessel wall.
2. A thrombus forms when blood components combine to form an aggregate body (clot).
3. Pulmonary embolism occurs when a clot traveling through the venous system lodges within the pulmonary circulatory system, causing occlusion or infarction.

**B.** **Etiology and pathophysiology**

1. The incidence of postpartum thrombophlebitis is 0.1% to 1%; when not treated, 24% of these develop pulmonary embolism, with a fatality rate of 15%.
2. Predisposing risk factors
   a. History of thrombophlebitis
   b. Obesity
   c. History of cesarean delivery

      d.   History of forceps delivery
      e.   Maternal age older than 35
      f.   Multiparity
      g.   Lactation suppression with estrogens
      h.   Varicosities
      i.   Anemia and blood dyscrasias

**C.**  **Assessment**

1. Superficial thrombophlebitis within the saphenous vein system manifests as midcalf pain, tenderness, redness along the vein.
2. Deep vein thrombosis (DVT) symptoms include muscle pain, positive Homans' sign (pain in the calf on passive dorsiflexion of the foot, possibly caused by DVT).
3. Pelvic thrombophlebitis, typically occurring 2 weeks after delivery, is marked by chills, fever, malaise, and pain.
4. Femoral thrombophlebitis, generally occurring 10 to 14 days after delivery, produces chills, fever, malaise, stiffness, and pain.
5. Pulmonary embolism is heralded by sudden intense chest pain with severe dyspnea followed by tachypnea, pleuritic pain, apprehension, cough, tachycardia, hemoptysis, and temperature above 38°C (100.4°F).

**D.**  **Nursing diagnoses**

1. Risk for Injury
2. Knowledge Deficit
3. Impaired Physical Mobility
4. Pain
5. Altered Parenting
6. Self Care Deficit

**E.**  **Planning and implementation**

1. Assess vital signs.
2. Assess extremities for signs of inflammation, swelling, positive Homans' sign.
3. Explain strategies for preventing venous stasis, such as:
    a.   Ambulating early and preventing pressure on legs
    b.   Avoiding standing or sitting for long periods of time
    c.   Avoiding crossing legs
4. Administer anticoagulant therapy as prescribed, and observe for signs of bleeding and allergic reactions.
5. **Keep the antidote protamine sulfate available in case of a severe heparin overdose. Usually, protamine sulfate solution is administered intravenously at a rate no greater than 50 mg/10 min.**
6. Caution: Do not administer estrogens for lactation suppression, because estrogens may encourage clot formation.

7. Prepare client for diagnostic studies (ie, venography and Doppler ultrasound) as indicated.
8. Implement measures to prevent complications of bed rest as needed (eg, bed placed in Trendelenburg position, use of footboard, passive or active range of motion exercises, frequent shifts in position, adequate fluid intake and output).
9. Support and communicate with client and family members during an emergency situation, thus enhancing cooperation with treatment efforts.
10. Provide information regarding treatment regimen (eg, anticoagulant therapy, analgesics, and bed rest).

F. **Evaluation**
1. The mother is pain free, breathes normally, and returns to stable condition.
2. The mother and family understand events and treatment.
3. The mother can continue care of self and newborn.

# VI. Urinary tract infection

A. **Description**
1. Bacteria defined as $>10^5$ bacterial colonies/mL of urine in two consecutive clean, voided, midstream specimens
2. Retention and residual urine: overdistention and incomplete emptying of bladder
3. Cystitis: inflammation of the urinary bladder
4. Pyelonephritis: inflammation of renal pelvis

B. **Etiology and pathophysiology**
1. Urinary tract infections occur in about 5% of postpartum women; they occur in 15% of women who have undergone postpartum catheterization.
2. Temporary urine retention may be due to decreased perception of the urge to void, resulting from perineal trauma and the effects of analgesia or anesthesia.
3. Urinary stasis and residual urine provide a medium for bacterial growth, predisposing the client to cystitis and pyelonephritis.
4. Causative organisms in cystitis and pyelonephritis include *E. coli* (most common), *Proteus, Pseudomonas, S. aureus,* and *Streptococcus faecalis.*
5. Consequences of not recognizing early symptoms include the extension of the infection upward with subsequent permanent loss of kidney function.

C. **Assessment**
1. Manifestations of cystitis include frequency, urgency, dysuria, hematuria, nocturia, temperature elevation, and suprapubic pain.

2. Symptoms of pyelonephritis include high fever, chills, flank pain, nausea, and vomiting.

**D. Nursing diagnoses**

1. Risk for Injury
2. Pain
3. Urinary Retention

**E. Planning and implementation**

1. Obtain specimens, report findings, and administer antibiotics and medications as prescribed.
2. Insert intermittent or indwelling catheter as needed.
3. Observe and record response to treatment.
4. Determine if symptoms are present and if woman had difficulty urinating after delivery.
5. Describe self-care related to regular emptying of bladder, proper perineal cleansing, and the need for increased fluids.

**F. Evaluation**

1. The mother can void and empty bladder.
2. The mother can care for self.
3. The mother can follow through with treatment plan.
4. The mother's urine bacteria colony count decreases to within normal range, and symptoms subside.

## VII. Postpartum mood disorders

**A. Description: also called postpartum blues, postpartum depression, or postpartum psychosis, puerperal mental or emotional problems may be manifest in various symptoms, but all have postpartum onset in common.**

**B. Etiology and pathophysiology**

1. Between **50% and 80% of all new mothers report some form of postpartum "blues."**
2. Incidence of moderate or major postpartum depression or postpartum bipolar disorder ranges from 30 to 200 per every 1,000 live births; incidence of brief psychotic disorder with postpartum onset is about 1 in every 1,000 live births.
3. Predisposing factors include history of puerperal psychosis, bipolar (formerly manic-depressive) disorder, delirium and hallucinations, rapid mood changes, agitation or confusion, potential for suicide or infanticide.

**C. Assessment**

1. Symptoms associated with postpartum depression include confusion, fatigue, agitation, feelings of hopelessness and shame, and alterations in mood. Additional symptoms of a major mood disorder include depression, ambivalence about the pregnancy, feelings of inadequacy, marital discord, guilt, and irritability.

2. Findings and client complaints associated with psychosis include delusions, auditory hallucinations, and hyperactivity.
3. Serious postpartum depression or psychosis usually does not occur until 3 to 5 days after delivery, at which time the client is usually discharged from the hospital or birthing center.

**D. Nursing diagnoses**
1. Anxiety
2. Ineffective Individual Coping
3. Ineffective Family Coping: Compromised
4. Altered Family Processes
5. Altered Parenting

**E. Planning and implementation**
1. Plan for continuity of care for mother, newborn, and family.
2. Develop specific therapeutic goals.
3. Maintain the prescribed medication schedule.
4. Provide support for mother's continued care of newborn if appropriate and safe for newborn.
5. Keep communication open with health care providers; coordinate social services.
6. Include family participation and involvement in plans for care.
7. Make appropriate referrals.

**F. Evaluation**
1. The mother is free of symptoms.
2. The mother can maintain a healthy relationship with the newborn and family.
3. The mother assumes responsibility for care of newborn and herself.

## Bibliography

American Psychiatric Association (1994). *Diagnostic and statistical manual-IV*. Washington, DC: Author.

Bobak, I. M., & Jensen, M. D. (1993). *Maternity and gynecologic care: The nurse and the family* (5th ed.). St. Louis: C.V. Mosby.

Johnson, B. S. (1994). *Child, adolescent, and family psychiatric nursing*. Philadelphia: J.B. Lippincott.

May, K. A., & Mahlmeister, L. R. (1994). *Maternal and neonatal nursing: Family-centered care* (3rd ed.). Philadelphia: J.B. Lippincott.

Olds, S. B., London, M. L., & Ladewig, P. W. (1992). *Maternal-newborn nursing: A family centered approach* (4th ed.). Menlo Park, CA: Addison-Wesley.

Reeder, S. J., Martin, L. L., & Koniak, D. (1992). *Maternity nursing: Family newborn, and women's health care* (17th ed.). Philadelphia: J.B. Lippincott.

# STUDY QUESTIONS

1. With today's short postpartum hospitalizations (24–72 hours), the focus of nursing revolves around which of the following essential concepts?
   a. To promote comfort and recovery through physical care measures and pain relief therapies
   b. To explore the emotional aspects of care of the high-risk newborn and the family
   c. To assist parents to care for themselves and their newborn safely and effectively
   d. To assist the client and family to deal with anxiety effectively

2. The overall nursing objectives for high-risk postpartum clients include which of the following factors?
   a. Implementing self-care for the mother and her newborn and discussing hygiene and nutrition
   b. Referring the mother to others for emotional support to minimize postpartum depression
   c. Asking the physician to discuss complications, expected course, and treatment
   d. Implementing routine nursing procedures and promoting mother–newborn contact

3. From the following, select the amount of blood loss that marks the criterion for describing postpartum hemorrhage.
   a. Blood loss of more than 500 mL following birth
   b. Blood loss of more than 400 mL following birth
   c. Blood loss of more than 300 mL following birth
   d. Blood loss of more than 200 mL following birth

4. Identify the best description of subinvolution.
   a. It occurs in the first 24 hours after delivery and contains fragments of placental tissue.
   b. It is delayed healing, resulting from retained placental fragments, membranes, and endometritis.
   c. It occurs in the first 8 hours after birth; the discharge contains fragments of placental tissue.
   d. It is the result of difficult labor and traumatic delivery of the placenta.

5. From the following statements, select the one that best signals early puerperal infection.
   a. It is marked by temperature elevation of 38°C (100.4°F) or higher after the first 24 postpartum hours.
   b. It is marked by local infections of the vagina, vulva, and perineum after the first 24 postpartum hours.
   c. It is characterized by elevated temperature, dyspnea, hypovolemia, and malaise after the first 12 postpartum hours.
   d. It is characterized by lower abdominal pain, inability to void, and anxiety following the first postpartum week.

6. Which of the following is the *primary* predisposing factor related to mastitis?
   a. Epidemic infection that comes from nosocomial sources and localizes in the lactiferous glands and ducts
   b. Endemic infection occurring randomly and localizing in the periglandular connective tissue
   c. Infection that may appear at the end of the first postpartum week but most commonly in the third and fourth week
   d. Breast injury caused by overdistention, stasis, and cracking of the nipples

7. Which of the following best describes thrombophlebitis?
   a. Inflammation and clot formation that result when blood components combine to form an aggregate body
   b. Inflammation and blood clots that eventually become lodged within the pulmonary blood vessels

c. Inflammation and blood clots that eventually become lodged within the vessels that nourish the uterus

d. Inflammation of the vascular endothelium with clot formation on the vessel wall

8. Which of the following assessment findings would appear with DVT?
   a. Midcalf pain, tenderness, and redness along the vein
   b. Chills, fever, malaise, and depression occurring 2 weeks after delivery
   c. Muscle pain, positive Homans' sign, and swelling in the affected limb
   d. Chills, fever, malaise, stiffness, and pain occurring 10 to 14 days after delivery

9. Of the following groups of signs and symptoms, which includes the most commonly assessed findings in cystitis?
   a. Frequency, urgency, dehydration, albuminuria, and suprapubic pain
   b. Frequency, urgency, dysuria, hematuria, nocturia, fever, and suprapubic pain
   c. Dehydration, hypertension, dysuria, suprapubic pain, chills, and fever
   d. High fever, chills, flank pain, nausea, vomiting, dysuria, and frequency

10. Which of the following best reflects the frequency of reported postpartum "blues"?
    a. Between 10% and 40% of all new mothers report some form of postpartum blues.
    b. Between 30% and 50% of all new mothers report some form of postpartum blues.
    c. Between 50% and 80% of all new mothers report some form of postpartum blues.
    d. Between 25% and 70% of all new mothers report some form of postpartum blues.

# ANSWER KEY

**1.** *Correct response: c*
Today, relatively short postpartum hospitalizations (for most clients, 24–72 hours) require the nurse to focus postpartum care on assisting parents to care for themselves and their newborn safely and effectively.
a, b, and d. All of these are factors, but the overall situation should be the most important.
*Knowledge/Safe Care/Assessment*

**2.** *Correct response: d*
Overall nursing objectives for high-risk postpartum clients include all of the routine objectives, plus minimizing the separation of mother and newborn and encouraging attachment.
a. This is true but should be considered as one of the general activities.
b and c. These are nursing responsibilities and should not be passed over or referred to others.
*Knowledge/Psychosocial/Implementation*

**3.** *Correct response: a*
Postpartum hemorrhage is blood loss of more than 500 mL following birth.
b, c, and d. All are incorrect answers.
*Knowledge/Physiologic/Assessment*

**4.** *Correct response: b*
Subinvolution results from retained placental fragments and membranes or endometritis.
a and c. These are incorrect answers.
d. Hemorrhage would occur at the time of placental removal or soon after.
*Knowledge/Physiologic/NA*

**5.** *Correct response: a*
Puerperal morbidity is marked by temperature elevation of 38°C (100.4°F) or higher after the first 24 postpartum hours on any 2 of the first 10 postpartum days.
b, c, and d. All may be present with peurperal infection, but the temperature elevation is usually the first definitive sign.
*Comprehension/Physiologic/Assessment*

**6.** *Correct response: d*
Injury to the breast is the primary predisposing factor (eg, overdistention, stasis, cracking of the nipples).
a and b. These are probable sources of infection.
c. This statement describes a symptom not a predisposing factor.
*Knowledge/Safe Care/Assessment*

**7.** *Correct response: d*
Thrombophlebitis is an inflammation of the vascular endothelium with clot formation on the wall of the vessel.
a. This describes a thrombus or thrombosis.
b. This describes pulmonary embolism.
c. This is incorrect.
*Knowledge/Physiologic/NA*

**8.** *Correct response: c*
Classic symptoms of DVT include muscle pain, positive Homans' sign, and swelling of the affected limb.
a. These symptoms reflect superficial thrombophlebitis.
b. These symptoms reflect pelvic thrombophlebitis.
d. These symptoms reflect femoral thrombophlebitis.
*Comprehension/Safe Care/Assessment*

**9.** *Correct response: b*
Manifestations of cystitis include frequency, urgency, dysuria, hematuria nocturia, fever, and suprapubic pain.
a. This is only partially correct.
c. This is incorrect.
d. These findings reflect pyelonephritis.
*Knowledge/Physiologic/Assessment*

**10.** *Correct response: c*
Between 50% and 80% of all new mothers report some form of postpartum blues.
a, b, and d. All are incorrect percentages.
*Knowledge/Physiologic/Assessment*

# Neonatal Complications

## I. Overview

### A. Essential concepts

1. Early identification of the high-risk newborn is the first step in detecting and managing complications to reduce morbidity and mortality.

2. Major neonatal complications covered in this chapter include:
   a. Birth asphyxia

    b.    Complications related to gestational age: preterm, small for gestational age (SGA), large for gestational age (LGA), post-term

    c.    Complications related to maternal condition (eg, diabetes)

**3.**    Complications not covered extensively in this chapter include:

    a.    Birth injuries (eg, fractures of skull, clavicle, humerus, or femur)

    b.    Infection: bacterial, viral, protozoal

    c.    Hemolytic disease: Rh and ABO incompatibility

    d.    Central nervous system injuries (eg, intracranial hemorrhage, brachial plexus injury, facial nerve injury, phrenic nerve injury)

    e.    Maternal substance abuse (eg, alcohol and other drugs)

**B.**    **General nursing management of the high-risk newborn**

**1.**    Assessment: Components include maternal and neonatal health histories, systematic physical and behavioral assessments, screening for risk factors, and ongoing assessments of high-risk conditions, for example:

    a.    Alcohol use: Because the safe amount of alcohol use remains unknown, newborns of mothers who use alcohol are at risk for fetal alcohol syndrome (FAS). Classic effects of FAS include:

        ► Intrauterine growth retardation
        ► Mental retardation
        ► Neurologic damage
        ► Congenital deformities
        ► Microcephaly

    b.    Other drugs (eg, narcotics, cocaine, nicotine): The newborn of a mother who is dependent on prescription or nonprescription substances may experience complications requiring emergency measures. Complications include:

        ► Neurologic problems, such as reflex irritability, tremors, and possibly seizures
        ► Respiratory compromise and apnea
        ► GI symptoms, such as poor feeding, regurgitation, projectile vomiting, and airway obstruction

**2.**    Nursing diagnoses: In addition to complication-specific nursing diagnoses, the following diagnoses are common to care of high-risk newborns:

    a.    Risk for Altered Body Temperature

    b.    Fluid Volume Deficit

    c.    Impaired Gas Exchange

    d.    Risk for Infection

      e.    Altered Nutrition: Less than body requirements

      f.    Altered Parenting

**3.**   Planning and implementation

      a.    Support cardiopulmonary adaptation; maintain adequate airway.

      b.    Administer oxygen using oxygen mask, endotracheal tube, oxygen hood, or nasal prongs.

      c.    Support ventilatory capacity.

      d.    Promote fluid and electrolyte balance.

      e.    Maintain adequate nutrition.

      f.    Prevent infection

      g.    Support thermoregulation.

      h.    Promote behavioral adaptation and parent–newborn attachment.

      i.    Screen for potential complications related to oxygen toxicity (eg, retinopathy of prematurity and bronchopulmonary dysplasia).

      j.    Observe for the potential complications of hyperbilirubinemia and kernicterus.

      k.    Support conjugation and excretion of bilirubin.

      l.    Initiate phototherapy as necessary.

         ▶  Position the naked newborn 18 in from light source, cover his or her eyes, and avoid using oils or lotions that may cause burns.

         ▶  Turn the newborn every 2 hours.

      m.   Evaluate the possibility of altered parenting.

**4.**   Evaluation

      a.    The newborn achieves and maintains normal cardiac output and adequate tissue perfusion.

      b.    The newborn exhibits and maintains normal respiratory pattern and adequate gas exchange.

      c.    The newborn achieves fluid and electrolyte balance.

      d.    Nutritional requirements for growth and development are maintained.

      e.    The newborn remains free of infection.

      f.    The newborn maintains normal core temperature.

      g.    The newborn achieves a state of behavioral stabilization and beginning organization.

      h.    The newborn undergoing oxygen therapy has no oxygen toxicity.

      i.    The newborn undergoing phototherapy responds with reduced hyperbilirubinemia.

      j.    The newborn receiving exchange transfusion remains free of complications and maintains serum bilirubin levels within normal limits.

## II. Birth asphyxia

240

**A.** Description: a condition characterized by hypoxemia (decreased $PaO_2$), hypercarbia (increased $PaCO_2$), and acidosis (lowered pH)

**B.** Etiology and incidence

1. Causes
   a. Impaired maternal blood flow through the placenta
   b. Impaired blood flow through the umbilical cord
   c. Impaired fetal circulation
   d. Impaired respiratory effort
2. Unless vigorous resuscitation begins promptly, irreversible changes in brain and myocardial tissues will occur, possibly leading to permanent brain damage or death.
3. **During the 24 hours after successful resuscitation, the newborn is vulnerable to postasphyxial syndrome.**

**C.** Assessment

1. Clinical signs of birth asphyxia include:
   a. Decreased $PaO_2$ level
   b. Increased $PaCO_2$
   c. Low pH
   d. Minimal or absent respiratory effort
   e. Depressed cardiac function
2. The newborn may gasp for breath in an attempt to inflate the lungs.

**D.** Nursing diagnoses

1. Ineffective Breathing Pattern
2. Impaired Gas Exchange

**E.** Planning and implementation

1. Observe newborn who has been successfully resuscitated for the following constellation of signs:
   a. Seizure activity in the first 24 hours after birth
   b. Necrosis of renal and intestinal tissues
   c. Metabolic alterations (eg, hypoglycemia, hypocalcemia, hyperkalemia)
   d. Increased intracranial pressure marked by bulging fontanels, "setting sun" eyes, decreased or absent reflexes, and seizures
   e. Myocardial ischemia (arrhythmias), intestinal ischemia, and necrotizing enterocolitis (NEC), which is the absence of bowel sounds, increasing abdominal girth, and bloody stools
2. Maintain the intestinal tract in a resting state by giving the newborn nothing by mouth for 24 to 48 hours.

3. Measure and record intake and output to evaluate renal function.
4. Check every voiding for blood and protein, suggesting renal injury.
5. Check every stool for blood, suggesting NEC.
6. Facilitate serial blood glucose determinations to detect hypoglycemia and serum electrolytes, as ordered.
7. Administer and maintain intravenous fluids.
8. Administer antibiotics and seizure medications (eg, phenytoin, phenobarbital) as prescribed.
9. Maintain neutral thermal environment.
10. Support parents in dealing with the seriousness of the event.
11. Administer oxygen as needed.

**F. Evaluation**

1. Complications of postasphyxial syndrome are identified early and appropriate interventions maintained.
2. Newborn responds to treatment for seizure activity, as evidenced by normalization of neurologic and physiologic status and absence of recurrent seizure activity.
3. Parents verbalize accurate understanding of the newborn's condition and prognosis.

## III. Preterm newborn

**A. Description: newborn born before 37 weeks' gestation**

**B. Etiology and pathophysiology**

1. The etiology of preterm labor is poorly understood.
2. Among the many possible factors are:
   a. Premature rupture of the membranes
   b. Preeclampsia
   c. Hydramnios
   d. Placenta previa
   e. Abruptio placentae
   f. Incompetent cervix
   g. Trauma
   h. Uterine structural anomalies
   i. Congenital adrenal hyperplasia
   j. Fetal death

3. **Maternal risk factors include age less than 18 years, history of preterm labors, multiple pregnancy, hydramnios, smoking, poor hygiene, poor nutrition, employment.**
4. Preterm newborns exhibit anatomic and physiologic immaturity in all body systems; this immaturity hinders the adaptations to extrauterine life that the newborn must make.

**C.** **Assessment**

1. Respiratory status: tachypnea, grunting, nasal flaring, retractions, cyanosis
2. Cardiovascular status: decreased oxygen saturation, decreased oxygen levels, abnormal arterial blood gas (ABG) values
3. Gastrointestinal status: decreased gag, suck, and swallow reflexes; gastric reflux; vomiting; gastric residuals; weight loss; failure to gain 10 to 15 g/d
4. Fluid status
   a. Fluid excess: edema, congestive heart failure
   b. Fluid deficit: tachycardia, poor skin turgor, decreased urine output, abnormal electrolyte levels, increased urine osmolarity (pH), decreased blood pressure
5. Physiologic anemia: tachycardia, pallor, decreased blood pressure, apnea, failure to gain weight
6. Signs and symptoms of neonatal infection: temperature instability, apnea, cyanosis, decreased oxygen saturation, poor feeding, gastric residuals
7. Hypoglycemia or hyperglycemia
8. Temperature control: unstable body core temperature
9. Neuromuscular system status: arching behaviors, hyperextension of extremities, resistance to cuddling
10. Altered parenting:
    a. Decreased or absent parental visits
    b. Parental resistance or refusal to participate in newborn care
    c. Denial of severity of newborn illness
    d. Resistance or refusal to touch newborn
    e. Persistent verbalization of guilt

**D.** **Nursing diagnoses**

1. Ineffective Airway Clearance
2. Ineffective Breathing Patterns
3. Fluid Volume Excess or Fluid Volume Deficit
4. Impaired Gas Exchange
5. Hypothermia
6. Risk for Infection
7. Impaired Physical Mobility
8. Altered Nutrition: Less than body requirements
9. Altered Parenting

**E.** **Planning and implementation**

1. Maintain a patent airway:
   a. Suction the newborn as indicated.
   b. Maintain the airway by positioning the newborn on his or her side or on the back with a thin (1 in or less) rolled washcloth under the shoulders.

    c.    As needed, reposition the newborn to help drain mucus or regurgitated milk.

**2.** Support respiratory efforts:

    a.    Electronically monitor breathing and heart rate.

    b.    Prevent gastric distention by aspirating air before gavage feedings and by avoiding overfeeding.

    c.    **Discontinue oral feeding if respiratory distress occurs.**

    d.    Administer oxygen to keep $PaO_2$ between 50 and 80 mm Hg on ABG analysis.

**3.** Monitor ambient oxygen concentration with an oxygen analyzer; use a noninvasive $TcPO_2$ monitor or an oxygen saturation monitor (pulse oximeter).

**4.** Provide appropriate nutrition.

    a.    Administer formula as prescribed.

    b.    Position the newborn on the right side after feeding to promote stomach emptying.

    c.    Avoid disturbing the newborn for at least 1 hour after feeding to facilitate stomach emptying and nutrient absorption.

**5.** Evaluate for evidence of exhaustion during feeding.

    a.    Maintain neutral thermal environment and normal body temperature.

    b.    Evaluate respiratory effort during feeding.

    c.    Weigh newborn daily, and plot growth on chart.

**6.** Observe for development of life-threatening NEC.

    a.    Check residual gastric content (gastric residuals) before feeding, and report an increasing or a sudden large volume of residual.

    b.    Measure abdominal girth every 4 hours.

    c.    Document any vomiting; note frequency and characteristics of emesis, including color, odor, and amount.

**7.** Monitor for fluid volume excess:

    a.    Precisely measure intake and output.

    b.    Administer diuretics as prescribed.

    c.    Regulate all intravenous infusions with an intravenous infusion pump.

    d.    Administer other solutions and formulas as prescribed.

**8.** Prevent fluid volume excess or deficit:

    a.    Assess daily sodium, chloride, and potassium levels.

    b.    Minimize insensible water losses; cover the newborn with a heat shield, humidify oxygen, and close isolette ports.

    c.    Minimize withdrawal of blood for laboratory analysis.

    d.    Test all voidings for pH and specific gravity.

**9.** Prevent physiologic anemia:

    a.    Minimize withdrawal of blood for laboratory analysis.

       b.   Administer vitamin K to prevent hemorrhagic disease of the newborn.

       c.   Place the newborn in a neutral thermal environment to decrease energy requirements in case of severe anemia.

10.   Detect early metabolic changes by testing blood glucose levels with a reagent strip, such as Dextrostix or Chemstrip.

11.   Prevent hypothermia and cold stress by placing the newborn in a neutral thermal environment.

12.   Observe for skin jaundice and signs and symptoms of bilirubin encephalopathy.

13.   Encourage flexion in the supine position by using blanket rolls.

14.   Provide the newborn with body boundaries through swaddling or using blanket rolls against the newborn's body and feet.

15.   Develop an appropriate newborn stimulation plan based on gestational age, physiologic limitations, and presence of disease.

16.   Observe for altered parenting, and facilitate parental attachment:

       a.   Encourage early and frequent visits by parents.

       b.   Place name on newborn's isolette.

       c.   Provide parents with the unit phone number and names of staff caring for the newborn.

       d.   Give parents the opportunity to provide progressively complex care for the newborn.

       e.   Point out the newborn's unique characteristics.

**F.**   **Evaluation**

1.   The preterm newborn establishes respiratory function, as evidenced by successful weaning from mechanical support by the time of discharge.

2.   The preterm newborn gains weight and shows no signs of gastrointestinal complications.

3.   The preterm newborn achieves fluid and electrolyte balance, as evidenced by output of 1 to 3 mL/kg per hour in the first week of life.

4.   The preterm newborn maintains hematocrit level of 10 g/dL.

5.   The preterm newborn remains free of metabolic alterations.

6.   The preterm newborn maintains a normal core temperature, as evidenced by axillary temperature of 36.4°C to 37.2°C.

7.   The preterm newborn remains free of hyperbilirubinemia or encephalopathy.

8.   The preterm newborn develops increasingly organized patterns of behavior and demonstrates age-appropriate growth and development.

9.   Parents of the preterm newborn demonstrate appropriate and progressive attachment behaviors (eg, frequent visits or calls,

increasing interest and confidence in providing care, calling the newborn by name).

## IV. SGA newborn

**A.** Description: weighs less than most newborns, below the 10th percentile or 2 standard deviations below the mean, as a result of intrauterine growth retardation (IUGR)

**B.** Etiology and pathophysiology

1. Predisposing factors include maternal malnutrition, premature placental aging secondary to diabetes mellitus or other vascular conditions, placental infarcts, congenital infections, teratogens, and maternal substance abuse or cigarette smoking.

2. In symmetrical IUGR, the fetus experiences early and prolonged nutritional deprivation caused by severe, chronic maternal malnutrition; placental insufficiency; intrauterine infection; or fetal chromosomal anomalies. It is characterized by:
   a. Hypoplastic cell growth and development
   b. Head circumference below 10th percentile
   c. Diminished brain size and possible mental retardation

3. Asymmetrical IUGR results from nutritional deficits and placental insufficiency in late pregnancy. It is characterized by:
   a. Diminished cell size but not cell numbers
   b. Disproportionately large head in relation to body, with long and emaciated trunk and little subcutaneous fat
   c. Head circumference approaching normal

4. In asymmetrical IUGR, newborn growth and development are rapid, and the potential for normal intellectual functioning is excellent.

**C.** Assessment

1. Respiratory status and breathing pattern: tachypnea, grunting, flaring, retractions, cyanosis, decreased oxygen saturation, abnormal ABGs

2. Physical features and growth status: dysmorphic features; wasting of trunk and extremities; rough, dry skin; large anterior fontanel

3. Nutritional status: gastric reflux, weight loss, failure to gain weight (10–15 g/d)

4. Metabolic status: jitteriness, lethargy, cyanosis, apnea, blood glucose level 45 mg/dL or less

5. Hematologic status: hematocrit >65%, cyanosis, respiratory dis-

tress, central nervous system (CNS) aberrations (lethargy, poor feeding, convulsions, hypotonia)

6. Unstable temperature control: temperature swings, temperature 36.4°C or less

**D. Nursing diagnoses**
1. Ineffective Airway Clearance
2. Ineffective Breathing Pattern
3. Ineffective Gas Exchange
4. Altered Growth and Development
5. Hypothermia
6. Altered Nutrition: Less than body requirements

**E. Planning and implementation**
1. Support airway clearance by suctioning as needed, administering humidified mist to liquefy secretions, and performing chest physiotherapy to facilitate drainage.

2. **Electronically monitor cardiopulmonary status; position newborn to facilitate chest expansion and prevent stomach distention (eg, avoid overfeeding; aspirate air before gavage feeding).**

3. Promote effective gas exchange by administering oxygen to maintain $PaO_2$ at 60 to 80 mm Hg; monitor concentrations with a $PtCO_2$ monitor or $O_2$ monitor.

4. Assess prenatal history for possible toxoplasmosis, rubella, cytomegalovirus, and herpes simplex infections during pregnancy or maternal substance abuse; assess immunoglobulin M levels, which, if elevated, could indicate intrauterine infection.

5. Provide small, frequent feedings to accommodate the SGA newborn's small stomach capacity; obtain daily weights, and plot them on a growth chart.

6. Assess for evidence of hypoglycemia at birth, hourly until stable, and before feedings.

7. **Obtain central hematocrit at birth to evaluate for hyperviscosity; be alert for ischemia of organs, thrombus formation, hypoglycemia, and respiratory distress associated with polycythemia.**

8. Maintain a neutral thermal environment.

**F. Evaluation**
1. The SGA newborn maintains optimal respiratory and cardiac function.
2. The SGA newborn begins to gain weight and length and to approximate normal newborn parameters.
3. The SGA newborn maintains a normal core temperature.

**V.** **LGA newborn**

    **A.** Description: a newborn who weighs more than 4,000 g, is in the 90th percentile, or is 2 standard deviations above the mean

    **B.** Etiology and pathophysiology

        **1.** Predisposing factors include genetic predisposition, excessive maternal weight gain during pregnancy, maternal gestational diabetes.

        **2.** An infant of a diabetic mother (IDM) commonly is LGA due to high levels of maternal glucose that cross the placenta during pregnancy.

        **3.** An IDM with vascular changes also may be SGA due to decreased placental functioning.

        **4.** LGA newborns are at risk for:

            **a.** Hypoglycemia due to limited liver glycogen stores

            **b.** Polycythemia due to chronic intrauterine hypoxia, which causes increased red blood cell (RBC) production

            **c.** Birth injuries due to disproportionate size of newborn to birth passageway

            **d.** Hyperbilirubinemia due to breakdown of excess RBCs

    **C.** Assessment

        **1.** Prenatal history may reveal maternal diabetes mellitus.

        **2.** Examination may disclose signs and symptoms of hypoglycemia, such as blood glucose value of 45 mg/dL or less measured by reagent strip (Chemstrip), tremors, hypotonia, lethargy, irritability, apnea, seizures (relevant for SGA IDM as well).

        **3.** The LGA newborn is prone to complications of birth injury, such as:

            **a.** Fractured clavicle: crepitus, hematoma, or deformity over clavicle; decreased movement of arm on the affected side; asymmetrical or absent Moro reflex

            **b.** Bell's palsy: facial hemiparesis, evidenced by drooping of lip to normal side, no wrinkling of forehead on affected side

            **c.** Erb-Duchenne palsy or brachial plexus paralysis: one arm weakness or paralysis, weak or absent grip

            **d.** Phrenic nerve palsy: weakness of the diaphragm with possible dyspnea, decreased breath sounds in lower lobes, and poor to absent rise of the abdomen with inspiration

            **e.** Possible skull fracture: soft-tissue swelling over fracture site, visible indentation in scalp, cephalhematoma, positive skull x-ray, CNS signs with intracranial hemorrhage (eg, lethargy, seizures, apnea, hypotonia)

4.   Hyperthermia may result from increased amount of fatty tissue serving as insulation.

**D.   Nursing diagnoses**
1.   Altered Growth and Development
2.   Hyperthermia
3.   Risk for Injury

**E.   Planning and implementation**
1.   Assess for and prevent hypoglycemia:
     a.   Test blood glucose level by reagent strip (Dextrostix or Chemstrip) every 30 minutes four times, every hour until feedings are started, and then before each feeding until the newborn is stable.
     b.   Administer dextrose 5% in water ($D_5W$) by mouth using nipple or gavage.
     c.   Retest blood glucose level 30 minutes after feeding.
     d.   Notify the physician of decreased blood glucose readings.
     e.   Begin oral formula feeding or breast-feeding as soon as possible.
2.   If IDM, observe for potential complications (SGA, LGA, hypocalcemia, respiratory distress syndrome, polycythemia, undiagnosed congenital anomalies, or heart murmur).
3.   Observe for birth injury and complications.

**F.   Evaluation**
1.   The LGA newborn responds to appropriate support and demonstrates no signs of hypoglycemia.
2.   The LGA newborn makes the transition to extrauterine life without complications or with resolution of complications within a few days or weeks after birth.
3.   The LGA newborn maintains normal temperature.
4.   Parents of the LGA newborn demonstrate signs of growing attachment to the newborn by their participation in care and growing ease in handling the newborn.

## VI.   IDM

**A.   Description: may be SGA or LGA, with or without congenital anomalies and with or without birth injury**

**B.   Etiology and pathophysiology**
1.   In maternal hyperglycemia (eg, gestational diabetes mellitus or long-term diabetes *without* vascular changes):
     a.   Large amounts of amino acids, free fatty acids, and glucose are transferred to fetus.
     b.   Maternal insulin does not cross the placenta.
     c.   Fetal response to transferred substances:

> ▸ Islet cells of pancreas enlarge (hypertrophy).
> ▸ Hypertrophic cells produce large volumes of insulin, which acts as a growth hormone, and protein synthesis accelerates.
> ▸ Fat and glycogen are deposited in fetal tissue, and fetus grows large (macrosomia), especially if maternal blood glucose levels are not well controlled in the third trimester.

    d.   Various unknown factors also may contribute to changes.

2.   In maternal long-term diabetes *with* vascular changes, the newborn is usually SGA because of compromised placental blood flow, maternal hypertension, or pregnancy-induced hypertension, which restricts uteroplacental blood flow.

3.   Associated complications in IDM:

    a.   Fractures and nerve damage may occur from birth trauma.

    b.   Congenital anomalies (heart, kidney, vertebral, CNS) are three to five times more common, with incidence decreasing if maternal blood glucose levels remain controlled and normal in first trimester.

    c.   Risk for respiratory distress syndrome increases (high insulin levels interfere with production of pulmonary surfactant).

> ▸ **Lecithin/sphingomyelin (L/S) ratio may inaccurately produce lung maturity in the IDM (usually require L/S of 3:1 for IDM compared with L/S exceeding 2:1 for non-IDM).**
> ▸ Phosphatidylglycerol in amniotic fluid usually indicates that pulmonary surfactant, a factor in lung maturity, is adequate to support extrauterine respiration.

    d.   Hypoglycemia may result after birth from lack of glucose from mother but continued production of insulin by newborn.

    e.   Hypocalcemia may result from decreased parathyroid hormone production, especially if maternal diabetes is poorly controlled.

    f.   Polycythemia (hematocrit exceeding 65%) may result from decreased extracellular fluid and increased production of RBCs to meet oxygen needs of fetal life.

    g.   Organ damage may result from decreased blood flow and renal vein thrombosis.

    h.   **Hyperbilirubinemia may result from breakdown of excess RBCs after birth.**

**C.**   Assessment

1.   Congenital anomalies are more likely in IDMs who are SGA than in other SGA newborns.

2. Size differences and variations are more common in IDMs who are LGA than in other LGA newborns:
   a. Greater size results from fat deposits and hypertrophic liver, adrenals, and heart.
   b. All organs but brain are larger than normal.
   c. Length and head size are usually within normal range for gestational age (other LGA newborns tend to be longer with large heads).
3. Observation reveals characteristic appearance: round, red face; obese body; poor muscle in resting IDM. Newborn may be irritable and possibly tremulous when disturbed.
4. Possible signs and symptoms of hypoglycemia include jitteriness, irritability, diaphoresis (uncommon in normal newborn but may occur in IDM), blood glucose level less than 45 mg/dL.
5. Additional assessment (palpation and auscultation) may disclose congenital anomalies or fractures and other injuries.
6. Diagnostic testing may include:
   a. Blood glucose evaluation at 30 and 60 minutes and at 2, 4, 6, and 12 hours after birth as directed by nursery protocol:

   ▸ If results are abnormal, repeat testing every 30 to 60 minutes until newborn achieves stable level; also test before each feeding for 24 hours.
   ▸ If reagent strips indicate blood glucose levels less than 45 mg/dL, findings should be verified by laboratory and reported to pediatrician.

   ▸ **Hypoglycemia may be present but not apparent.**

D. **Nursing diagnoses**
   1. Risk for Disorganized Infant Behaviors
   2. Risk for Injury
   3. Fluid Volume Deficit
   4. Ineffective Breathing Pattern
   5. Ineffective Breastfeeding

E. **Planning and implementation**
   1. Establish initial data base.
   2. Review the mother's health history and history of the pregnancy.
   3. Complete initial newborn examination as newborn's condition permits.
   4. Measure newborn's glucose level according to nursery protocol.
   5. Administer intravenous fluids if prescribed.

 6. **Feed newborn early according to nursery protocol to pre-**

vent or treat hypoglycemia, which may be present but hidden and which may develop 1 to 2 hours after birth.

7. Watch for hypoglycemia manifest by irritability, tremors, diaphoresis, and low blood glucose. If these signs continue after feeding, observe for other complications.
8. If newborn cannot suck well or if respiratory rate exceeds normal (30–60 breaths per minute), initiate gavage feeding.
9. Obtain hematocrit value; report findings to physician.
10. Observe for signs of respiratory distress (nasal flaring, grunting, retractions, tachypnea).
11. Prevent cold stress, which increases metabolism, thereby consuming oxygen and glucose rapidly.
12. Explain newborn's need for close observation and frequent blood tests to parents.
13. Demonstrate and discuss newborn care.
14. Provide an opportunity for the mother to discuss her feelings and concerns.

### F. Evaluation

1. Newborn's blood glucose levels remain within normal limits.
2. Collaborative care required by newborn is given promptly and effectively.
3. The newborn remains free of further complications.
4. Newborn's mother expresses concerns and feelings openly.
5. Parents demonstrate effective care of newborn.

## VII. Post-term newborn

### A. Description: born after 42 weeks' gestation

### B. Etiology and pathophysiology

1. Factors associated with postmaturity include first pregnancies, grand multiparity, history of prolonged pregnancy, anencephaly, trisomy 16 to 18, and Seckel's dwarfism.
2. Mortality rate is twice that of full-term newborns.
3. The newborn is at increased risk for developing complications related to compromised uteroplacental perfusion and hypoxia (eg, meconium aspiration syndrome [MAS], pneumothorax, and potential complications of hypoglycemia, polycythemia, and hypothermia)

### C. Assessment

1. Characteristics include a long, thin newborn with wasted appearance, parchment-like skin, meconium-stained skin, nails, and umbilical cord as a result of intrauterine hypoxia.

2. **MAS is manifested by fetal hypoxia, meconium staining of amniotic fluid, respiratory distress at delivery, and meconium-stained vocal cords.**
3. The newborn may exhibit signs of pneumothorax: acute respi-

ratory distress (tachypnea, flaring, grunting, retraction), cyanosis or pallor, skin mottling, decreased $PaO_2$, asymmetrical chest expansion, possible diminished breath sounds on affected side, and cardiovascular changes.

**D.** **Nursing diagnoses**
1. Ineffective Breathing Pattern
2. Impaired Gas Exchange
3. Altered Growth and Development
4. Hypothermia

**E.** **Planning and implementation**

1. **When assisting with birth of a post-term newborn with meconium-stained amniotic fluid, be prepared to assist with tracheal suctioning, visualization of the cords, and respiratory support.**
   a. Initiate respiratory assistance using mechanical ventilation.
   b. Maintain a neutral thermal environment.
   c. Perform chest physiotherapy, postural drainage.
   d. Administer antibiotics as prescribed.
   e. Administer a vasodilator if indicated to correct pulmonary hypertension.
   f. Maintain extracorporeal membrane oxygenation if indicated to correct persistent pulmonary hypertension.

2. Focus ongoing care of an uncomplicated post-term newborn on observation and support of respiratory function and prevention of complications:
   a. Obtain serial blood glucose measurements.
   b. Provide early feeding to prevent hypoglycemia if not contraindicated by respiratory status.

3. Be prepared for emergency aspiration and chest tube insertion followed by continuous monitoring of respiratory status if pneumothorax occurs.

**F.** **Evaluation**
1. The post-term newborn progresses and stabilizes with no untoward sequelae.
2. Complications of postmaturity are identified early.
3. Prompt interventions support the newborn's transition to extrauterine life.
4. Sequelae resolve within a few days or weeks of birth.
5. Parents of the post-term newborn demonstrate understanding of their newborn's condition and care.

# Bibliography

Bobak, I. M., & Jensen, M. D. (1993). *Maternity and gynecologic care: the nurse and the family* (5th ed.). St. Louis: C.V. Mosby.

May, K. A., & Mahlmeister, L. R. (1994). *Maternal and neonatal nursing: Family-centered care* (3rd ed.). Philadelphia: J.B. Lippincott.

Olds, S. B., London, M. L., & Ladewig, P. W. (1992). *Maternal-newborn nursing: A family centered approach* (4th ed.). Menlo Park, CA: Addison-Wesley.

Reeder, S. J., Martin, L. L., & Koniak, D. (1992). *Maternity nursing: Family newborn, and women's health care* (17th ed.). Philadelphia: J.B. Lippincott.

Wong, D. L. (1994). *Whaley and Wong's nursing care of infants and children* (5th ed.). St. Louis: C.V. Mosby.

# STUDY QUESTIONS

1. Identify the most important concept related to all high-risk newborns.
   a. To support the high-risk newborn's cardiopulmonary adaptation by maintaining an adequate airway
   b. To identify and intervene early for any complications in the high-risk newborn to reduce morbidity and mortality
   c. To assess the high-risk newborn for any physical complications that will assist the parents with bonding
   d. To support the mother and significant others in their quest toward adaptation to the high-risk newborn

2. Select the nursing interventions that most closely reflect the purpose of planning and implementing care for all high-risk newborns.
   a. Giving sufficient oxygen through mask, nasal prongs, endotracheal tube, or oxygen hood to prevent cyanosis
   b. Arranging counseling to help the family with their adaptation and emotional concerns
   c. Supporting cardiopulmonary adaptation, promoting fluid and electrolyte balance, and preventing infection
   d. Offering encouragement and giving the mother and signicant others references related to the care and special needs of the newborn

3. From the following, select the best description of birth asphyxia:
   a. It is characterized by hyperoxemia, hypercarbia, and acidosis.
   b. It is characterized by hyperoxemia, hypercarbia, and ketosis.
   c. It is characterized by hypoxemia, hypocarbia, and ketosis.
   d. It is characterized by hypoxemia, hypercarbia, and acidosis.

4. When planning and implementating care for the newborn who has been successfully resuscitated, the nurse should observe for which of the following?
   a. Seizure activity, metabolic alterations, increased intracranial pressure, and myocardial ischemia
   b. Seizure activity, metabolic alterations, prolonged apnea, and myocardial ischemia
   c. Muscle flaccidity, metabolic alterations, decreased intracranial pressure, and necrosis of the bowel
   d. Muscle flaccidity, necrosis of the renal and intestinal tissues, and increased intracranial pressure

5. Identify the *best* description of a preterm newborn.
   a. The newborn who is born before 25 weeks' gestation
   b. The newborn who is born after 25 weeks' gestation
   c. The newborn who is born after 37 weeks' gestation
   d. The newborn who is born before 37 weeks' gestation

6. From the following, select the group of terms that best describes assessment findings in the preterm newborn.
   a. Tachypnea, decreased or absent parental visits, constant return to fetal position, hyperpnea
   b. Tachypnea, abnormal ABG values, decreased gag and suck reflexes, temperature instability, and resistance to cuddling
   c. Cyanosis, abnormal ABG values, unstable body core temperature, and increased gag and suck reflexes
   d. Hyperpnea, unstable body core temperature, bradycardia, cyanosis, and arching behaviors with hyperextension

7. Some characteristics of an SGA newborn include which of the following?
   a. A newborn of normal weight, whose mother shows signs and symptoms of malnutrition, substance abuse, or placental aging

b. A normal newborn with congenital infection, fetal chromosomal anomalies, and near normal head circumference

c. A newborn of low weight whose mother shows signs and symptoms of malnutrition, substance abuse, or placental aging

d. A small newborn of low weight with congenital anomalies, inability to cuddle, and severe cyanosis

8. When implementing supportive measures for airway clearance for the SGA newborn, the nurse would plan to:

a. assess for hypoglycemia and other complications, such as fractures and Bell's palsy

b. perform suctioning as needed and position the newborn to facilitate chest expansion

c. observe for hypercalcemia, respiratory distress, polycythemia, and altered parenting

d. provide chest physiotherapy before feedings, remove mucus, and assess for potential respiratory distress

9. Select the statement best reflecting assessment findings in the LGA newborn.

a. The LGA newborn is prone to birth injuries, such as fractured clavicle, Bell's palsy, Erb-Duchenne palsy, and possible skull fracture.

b. The LGA newborn is prone to hypothermia, increased breath sounds in the lower pulmonary lobes, and substernal respiratory grunts.

c. The LGA newborn is prone to hyperactivity, with muscle rigidity, irritability, and infrequent seizures.

d. The LGA newborn is prone to dysmorphic features, wasting of the trunk and extremities, rough dry skin, and a large anterior fontanel.

10. Select the best description of the post-term newborn.

a. A newborn born after 48 weeks' gestation

b. A newborn whose mother has diabetes

c. A newborn born after 42 weeks' gestation

d. A newborn whose mother has a history of substance abuse

For additional questions, see
*Lippincott's Self-Study Series* Software
Available at your bookstore

# ANSWER KEY

1. **Correct response: b**
   Early identification of complications in the high-risk newborn is the first step toward intervening to reduce morbidity and mortality.
   **a, c, and d.** All are related to planned interventions for the high-risk newborn.
   *Analysis/Physiologic/Assessment*

2. **Correct response: c**
   Care for all high-risk newborns should include supporting cardiopulmonary adaptation, promoting fluid and electrolyte balance, and preventing infection. These interventions increase the newborn's chances of survival.
   **a.** Giving sufficient oxygen is not precise; specific amount should be monitored.
   **b.** This meets only family needs.
   **d.** This needs to be accomplished only if newborn survives.
   *Knowledge/Safe Care/Implementation*

3. **Correct response: d**
   Birth asphyxia is a condition characterized by hypoxemia, hypercarbia, and acidosis.
   **a, b, and c.** All are incorrect answers.
   *Knowledge/Physiologic/NA*

4. **Correct response: a**
   Observe the newborn who has been successfully resuscitated for seizure activity, metabolic alterations, increased intracranial pressure, and myocardial ischemia.
   **b, c, and d.** All are incorrect answers.
   *Knowledge/Physiologic/Implementation*

5. **Correct response: d**
   The preterm newborn is born before 37 weeks' gestation.
   **a, b, c.** All are incorrect numbers of weeks' gestation.
   *Knowledge/NA/NA*

6. **Correct response: b**
   Tachypnea, abnormal ABG values, decreased gag and suck reflexes, temperature instability, and resistance to cuddling are all assessment findings.
   **a.** Constant return to fetal position is incorrect.
   **c and d.** Hyperpnea and increased gag and suck reflexes are not correct.
   *Application/Physiologic/Assessment*

7. **Correct response: c**
   Some characteristics of the SGA newborn could be maternal malnutrition, maternal substance abuse, premature placental aging, and maternal diabetes.
   **a.** An SGA newborn would not have normal weight.
   **b.** A newborn with these complications would not be a normal newborn.
   **d.** These are complications not characteristics.
   *Knowledge/Physiologic/Assessment*

8. **Correct response: b**
   Clearing the newborn's airway by suctioning as needed and positioning to facilitate chest expansion are key interventions for maintaining airway patency in an SGA newborn.
   **a, c, and d.** All are incorrect answers.
   *Application/Physiologic/Implementation*

9. **Correct response: a**
   The LGA newborn is prone to birth injuries, such as fractured clavicle, palsy, Erb-Duchenne palsy, and possibly skull fracture.
   **b.** The LGA newborn is prone to hyperthermia.
   **c.** The LGA newborn is prone to lethargy and hypotonia.
   **d.** This is found in the post-term newborn.
   *Knowledge/Safe Care/Assessment*

10. **Correct response: c**
    The post-term newborn is born after 42 weeks' gestation.
    **a, b, and d.** All are incorrect numbers or maternal conditions.
    *Knowledge/NA/NA*

1. At 20 weeks' gestation, a primigravida client complains of swelling and pain in her "private area." On examination, you observe a red swollen area on the right side of the vaginal orifice. The client has an enlarged:
   a. Bartholin's gland
   b. clitoris
   c. parotid gland
   d. Skene's gland

2. The raised longitudinal folds of pigmented adipose tissue containing hair and extending from the mons veneris to the perineum is called the:
   a. labia minora
   b. labia majora
   c. mons pubis
   d. vestibule

3. The client's record indicates that she has a platypelloid pelvis. You know that this pelvis is:
   a. a typical female pelvis with rounded inlet
   b. a normal pelvis with heart-shaped inlet
   c. an apelike pelvis with an oval inlet
   d. a flat female pelvis with a transverse oval inlet

4. When examining the client's abdomen, you find that the tip of the uterus is 20 cm above the symphysis pubis. The upper rounded portion of the uterus is the:
   a. corpus
   b. decidua
   c. fundus
   d. isthmus

5. When measuring a woman's pelvic inlet, the obstetric conjugate is 10 cm. This indicates that the anteroposterior diameter is:
   a. within normal limits for a normal vaginal delivery
   b. too narrow for normal vaginal delivery
   c. extremely large
   d. marginal

6. If the embryo is to differentiate as a female, what hormonal stimulation must occur?
   a. An increase in maternal estrogen secretion
   b. A decrease in maternal androgen secretion
   c. Secretion of androgen by the fetal gonad
   d. Secretion of estrogen by the fetal gonad

7. A client is pregnant for the third time. She has a 3-year-old girl. She also has had a spontaneous abortion at 16 weeks' gestation. Which of the following is correct regarding gravida and para?
   a. Gravida 2, para 1
   b. Gravida 2, para 2
   c. Gravida 3, para 1
   d. Gravida 3, para 2

8. A new client has taken a pregnancy test to determine if she is pregnant. The hormone responsible for a positive pregnancy test result is:
   a. human chorionic gonadotropin
   b. estrogen
   c. follicle-stimulating hormone
   d. progesterone

9. A female client experiences amenorrhea, nausea, urinary frequency, and breast tenderness. These changes are known as:
   a. expected changes
   b. presumptive changes
   c. probable changes
   d. positive changes

10. During pelvic examination, the color of the client's cervix is blue-purple. This is called:
    a. Braxton's sign
    b. Chadwick's sign
    c. Goodell's sign
    d. McDonald's sign

11. A pregnant client complains of feeling faint while lying in a dorsal recumbent position. The nurse should:
    a. help the woman up into a sitting position

b. help the woman to turn on her left side in Sims' position
c. get the woman a drink of water
d. notify the physician immediately

12. While lying on the examination table during a prenatal check-up, a woman complains of a sudden grabbing pain in her calf muscle. Which of the following actions should the nurse take?
   a. Massage her calf.
   b. Place a warm compress on her calf.
   c. Dorsiflex her foot, and press her knee downward.
   d. Elevate her leg until the pain subsides.

13. The client says, "The doctor said there was ballottement present. What does this mean?" The nurse should explain that ballottement is the:
   a. examiner's palpation of contractions
   b. fetal movements felt by the mother
   c. passive movement of the unengaged fetus
   d. enlargement and softening of the uterus

14. The nurse examines a woman's breasts during a prenatal clinic visit. Which of the following findings must be reported to the physician?
   a. Tenderness
   b. Prominent superficial veins
   c. Increased pigmentation of areola and nipple
   d. Nodularity in the upper left outer quadrant

15. A pregnant client asks the nurse, "During this pregnancy, when will I gain the most weight?" The nurse's best response is:
   a. "Normally, weight is gained equally in each of the three trimesters."
   b. "Most weight is gained equally in the last two trimesters."
   c. "Most women gain too much in the first trimester and then try to decrease their gain in the second and third trimesters."
   d. "Most weight is gained (about 1 lb/wk) during the last two trimesters."

16. A woman asks, "The doctor wants me to have a sonogram next week. Why is this extra expense necessary?" The nurse's best response would be which of the following?
   a. "We want to determine the sex of the child so that you can plan for him or her."
   b. "It is important to determine the approximate date (within 2 weeks) of expected delivery."
   c. "This is a common practice due to the increasing number of lawsuits brought against obstetricians."
   d. "This is a way to diagnose early fetal anomalies."

17. A client reports that her only discomfort is slight nausea for part of the morning. Which of the following would be an inappropriate response by the nurse?
   a. "Bicarbonate of soda, 1 teaspoon in 8 oz of water, will decrease nausea."
   b. "Eating a few low-sodium crackers will often decrease the nausea."
   c. "Avoid liquid in the early morning."
   d. "Eating six smaller meals rather than three large meals will often decrease nausea."

18. A client asks if she can drink wine before going to sleep because wine helps her to relax. Which of the following would be the best response?
   a. "A couple of glasses a week would be all right."
   b. "It's best to avoid alcohol during pregnancy because a safe amount is not known."
   c. "Beer is safer to drink than wine."
   d. "Because you're entering your fourth month, it should be alright."

**19.** Breathing techniques are an important aspect of preparation for labor. Which of the following best describes the function of breathing techniques during labor?
   **a.** Breathing techniques can eliminate pain and will give the expectant parents something to do.
   **b.** Breathing techniques reduce the risk of fetal distress by increasing uteroplacental perfusion.
   **c.** Breathing techniques facilitate relaxation, require concentration, and may reduce the perception of pain.
   **d.** Breathing techniques can eliminate pain so that less analgesia and anesthesia are needed.

**20.** A couple is attending a childbirth class. They ask the nurse, "Why does back massage, especially pressure against the sacral area, soothe the woman during labor?" Which of the following would be the nurse's best response?
   **a.** "The pressure of massage counters the pressure from inside the woman and thereby eases her discomfort."
   **b.** "This pressure helps the baby rotate during its passage down the birth canal."
   **c.** "If the baby is in the posterior position, it helps the baby turn."
   **d.** "Lying in bed during labor makes the mother's back hurt."

**21.** The physician tells the nurse that a client has an android pelvis. The nurse asks if the client will have cesarean birth. The physician would most accurately respond with:
   **a.** "Android is a flat female pelvis."
   **b.** "She has a contracted pelvis, so she must be prepared for a cesarean birth."
   **c.** "Arrest of labor is common. A client with an android pelvis may require forceps manipulation or a cesarean birth."

   **d.** "You can tell the client there is no problem; she will have a vaginal delivery."

**22.** Of the various theories explaining the onset of labor, which of the following involves the release of a complex cascade of bioactive chemical agents into the amniotic fluid?
   **a.** Oxytocin theory
   **b.** Prostaglandin theory
   **c.** Progesterone deprivation theory
   **d.** Uterine decidua activation theory

**23.** A nurse who examines a client and finds a transverse lie may conclude which of the following?
   **a.** This is the woman's first baby.
   **b.** This woman has had two babies.
   **c.** This woman has a small uterus.
   **d.** This woman has pelvic contracture.

**24.** Which one of the following is *not* a sign of impending labor?
   **a.** Bloody show
   **b.** Rupture of membranes
   **c.** Back pain
   **d.** Patterned and rhythmic contractions

**25.** What stage of labor is the woman experiencing when she is in the active phase of labor?
   **a.** Stage one
   **b.** Stage two
   **c.** Stage three
   **d.** Stage four

**26.** A girl was born vaginally at 7:03 AM At 5 minutes, the heart rate is 100 beats/min; the cry is lusty with active motion of the extremities and a completely pink body. What is the 5-minute Apgar score for this newborn?
   **a.** 5
   **b.** 7
   **c.** 9
   **d.** 10

**27.** Following delivery, the newborn is placed in the radiant warmer to prevent hypothermia. Your first nursing action is to:

a. Cover the newborn with a warm blanket.
b. Place identification bands on the newborn.
c. Maintain respiration.
d. Administer vitamin K.

**28.** To promote drainage of mucus, place the newborn in which of the following positions to prevent airway blockage?
a. Sims' with shoulder roll
b. Trendelenburg
c. Lithotomy
d. Supine with shoulder roll

**29.** Shortly after delivery, you note that the mother's uterus is one finger breadth below the umbilicus and is displaced to the right of the abdomen. Your first priority would be to:
a. Assist the mother to void.
b. Vigorously massage the mother's fundus.
c. Administer an oxytocic drug.
d. Administer a tocolytic drug.

**30.** During the fourth stage of labor, the client asks, "Why do you keep pressing on my uterus? It sure is sore." You respond:
a. "I need to massage your fundus vigorously to prevent hemorrhage."
b. "It's important to check your uterus frequently to make sure you don't bleed too much."
c. "I realize it hurts, but it must be done."
d. "I'm following the doctor's orders."

**31.** You inform the client that right after delivery, the top of the uterus should feel:
a. firm, in the midline, and below the umbilicus
b. firm, to the right of the midline, and above the umbilicus
c. soft, in the midline, and at the umbilicus

d. soft, to the right of the midline, and above the umbilicus

**32.** A 26-year-old primigravida is admitted to the hospital in the active stage of labor. Four hours later, her contractions are not strong enough to cause the cervix to dilate, and uterine tone has decreased. Which of the following would you suspect?
a. Hypotonic uterine dysfunction related to ineffective contractions
b. Hypertonic uterine dysfunction related to ineffective contractions
c. Uterine dysfunction related to contracted pelvis
d. Uterine dysfunction related to maternal fatigue

**33.** When planning the same client's care, which of the following interventions would receive the highest priority?
a. Evaluation of blood loss
b. Evaluation of status of membranes
c. Evaluation of maternal and fetal vital signs
d. Evaluation of emotional status

**34.** The physician prescribes oxytocin administration by infusion pump. When monitoring the augmentation of labor, which nursing action would receive the highest priority?
a. Assessment of maternal vital signs
b. Assessment of fetal heart rate
c. Assessment of urinary output
d. Assessment of contractions for frequency, duration, and intensity

**35.** A 29-year-old multigravida at 38 weeks' gestation is admitted to the hospital with painless, bright red bleeding and mild contractions every 7 to 10 minutes. Which of the following assessments will the nurse avoid?
a. Assessment of maternal vital signs
b. Assessment of fetal heart rate
c. Assessment of contractions
d. Assessment of cervical dilation

**36.** Vaginal bleeding during the intrapartum period creates a high-risk situation. Base your thinking on the previous client's symptoms. Which of the following conditions would the client most likely have?

a. Abruptio placentae
b. Bloody show
c. Ectopic pregnancy
d. Placenta previa

37. To determine fetal status continuously during this client's labor, the nurse will assess fetal heart rate with:

a. a stethoscope
b. a fetoscope
c. an external monitor
d. an internal monitor

38. When caring for this client during labor, the nurse should be particularly alert for:

a. decreased urine output
b. anxiety and fatigue
c. discomfort with contractions
d. hemorrhage

39. The physician tells the client that she has a complete placenta previa and will need to have a cesarean birth. The client becomes wide eyed and begins to cry. She asks, "Why do I need to have a cesarean?" Which of the following would be the best response?

a. "Ask your physician when he returns."
b. "You need a cesarean to prevent hemorrhage."
c. "The placenta is covering 75% of the internal cervical os, and the baby cannot be delivered vaginally."
d. "The placenta is completely covering the opening of the uterus, so the baby cannot be delivered vaginally."

40. A fetus in a horizontal rather than a vertical plane is known to be positioned in a transverse lie. Which of the following could be the reason for this position?

a. Placenta previa
b. Abruptio placentae
c. Posterior fundal placenta attachment

d. Anterior fundal placenta attachment

41. If the client has been in true labor for 12 hours, and she has been diagnosed as having borderline pelvic measurements, the nurse should prepare for which of the following procedures?

a. Ultrasonography
b. Cesarean delivery
c. Radiographic pelvimetry
d. Manual internal pelvic measurement

42. A 42-year-old primipara client is both excited and concerned about her pregnancy. She is a candidate for prenatal diagnosis because of her age. Amniocentesis for prenatal diagnosis of genetic defects is usually done during which period of gestation?

a. 8 to 10 weeks
b. 14 to 16 weeks
c. 26 to 28 weeks
d. 32 to 34 weeks

43. A girl is delivered by cesarean section. Her diabetic mother experienced "good control" for 6 years before and during pregnancy. The plan of care for this newborn should include assessments for which of the following conditions?

a. Jaundice, hydrocephalus, and seizures
b. Large for gestational age, inability to maintain body temperature, and enlarged brain
c. Congenital anomalies, hemangioma, and mongolian spots
d. Excessive weight, respiratory distress, and tremors

44. A client was diagnosed as having diabetes mellitus when she was 12 years old. She is in her 36th week of pregnancy. Her insulin and diet have been closely regulated throughout her pregnancy. The physician orders several tests to measure fetal well-being. When comparing the results with previous ones, which of the following

would the nurse report to the physician immediately?

a. Decreased urine estriol
b. Decreased bilirubin
c. Increased creatinine
d. Increased lecithin-sphingomyelin ratio

**45.** This same client has progressed through pregnancy well. At 36 weeks' gestation, following several tests of fetal well-being, her primary care provider decides that labor can be induced early. What could be the rationale for this decision?

a. At term, the pregnant diabetic client is at increased risk for infection.
b. If allowed to go to term, the diabetic newborn tends to be large, leading to cephalopelvic disproportion.
c. The risk of severe hypoglycemic crisis during labor increases for the pregnant diabetic client near term.
d. The placenta of a diabetic mother tends to degenerate early, causing fetal distress.

**46.** A 32-year-old multipara had a cesarean delivery at 39 weeks' gestation secondary to an active herpesvirus type II infection. The client had pustular lesions on her vulva. When preparing the client for discharge, which of the following should the nurse include when discussing home care of mother and newborn?

a. The proper way to provide fundal massage for a relaxed uterus
b. Proper technique for scrubbing hands and gowning
c. The importance of bed rest for 1 week to avoid fatigue
d. The necessity of having someone else care for the newborn

**47.** Most elevated temperatures that occur in the first 24 postpartum hours are due to which of the following?

a. Dehydration
b. Breast engorgement

c. Vaginal infection
d. Uterine infection

**48.** If a new mother is in labor for 30 hours and her membranes are ruptured for 24 of the 30 hours, which of the following complications may occur?

a. Endometritis
b. Endometriosis
c. Salpingitis
d. Pelvic thrombophlebitis

**49.** Which of the following conditions would alert the nurse to possible postpartum hemorrhage?

a. Long labor and birth of twins
b. Cesarean birth
c. Premature birth
d. Dysfunctional labor and birth

**50.** Postpartum psychosis is a rare phenomenon but does occur. Which one of the following client behaviors would alert the nurse to the possibility of this occurrence?

a. Displaying great excitement about the birth experience
b. Crying spells in the early postpartum period
c. Complaining that fatigue prevents her from wanting to care for her newborn
d. Asking for pain medication and complaining of pain more than usual

**51.** A primigravida has delivered a 6-lb, 8-oz newborn 8 hours ago. When assessing this client, which of the following findings would require nursing intervention?

a. Temperature of 37.9°C (100.2°F)
b. Pulse rate of 60 beats/min
c. Perineal pad soaked with clots every 20 minutes
d. Excessive urination

**52.** If the fundus is above the umbilicus and shifts to one side, what should be the first nursing activity?

a. Check first for a full bladder.
b. Massage the uterus.

c. Suspect retained placental fragments.

d. Suspect clots in the uterus.

**53.** In the newborn of a narcotic-addicted mother, which of the following behaviors would be unusual?

a. Poor feeding

b. Tremors

c. High-pitched cry

d. Decreased reflex irritability

**54.** Characteristics of the newborn with fetal alcohol syndrome include which of the following?

a. A large head

b. Shorter length than usual for a full-term newborn

c. A smaller body and head

d. Heart defects

**55.** The nurse notices that a newborn is becoming jaundiced 12 hours after birth. Which would be the best nursing action?

a. Reassure the mother that this is physiologic jaundice and is normal.

b. This is not normal, and bilirubin blood levels should be assessed.

c. The mother is breast-feeding, and this is normal.

d. Alert the mother that the newborn may need an exchange transfusion.

**56.** A 20-year-old gravida 2, para 1 at 18 weeks' gestation is seen in the prenatal clinic for her second visit. Doppler assessment reveals fetal heart rate, 144; no edema; urine protein analysis, negative; weight, 124 lb; blood pressure, 112/72; temperature, 98°F; pulse, 84; respirations, 18; venereal disease research laboratory test (VDRL), negative; hemoglobin, 10 g/dL; and hematocrit, 32%. The client says, "I've been extremely tired and have had several dizzy spells." The nurse's best response would be:

a. "Tiredness and dizziness are normal during early pregnancy."

b. "Your laboratory findings and vital signs are within the normal range."

c. "Your hemoglobin is low, which could cause these symptoms."

d. "You are developing preeclampsia."

**57.** A 24-year-old gravida 1, para 0, insulin-dependent diabetic is seen in the clinic at 24 weeks' gestation. She states that the physician told her that her newborn is at risk because of her diabetes. She asks, "What does this mean?" The nurse should respond:

a. "The baby will not grow properly and is likely to be small."

b. "The baby will probably be a diabetic."

c. "Ask your doctor what she meant."

d. "There is a possibility of special problems and early labor."

**58.** The same client asks, "Will my insulin dosage be the same while I'm pregnant?" From the following, select the nurse's best response:

a. "Only if your doctor recommends a change when you have your regular office appointment."

b. "Your insulin may be the same. Why not call your obstetrician and talk it over?"

c. "You may experience some insulin resistance from hormonal changes."

d. "Your doctor will check your blood glucose level and adjust your insulin dosage if needed during your routine visits."

**59.** When gathering assessment data, the nurse learns that the client has a cardiac problem as a result of rheumatic fever. Which of the following statements best indicates that the client understands the danger signs of congestive heart failure?

a. "I should report pigmentation changes."

b. "I should report a frequent cough."

c. "I should report progressive fatigue."

d. "I should report colostrum."

60. The client in the previous situation asks, "When will I most likely develop heart problems during my pregnancy?" The nurse should respond that signs of cardiac complications generally become apparent at:
a. 14 to 18 weeks' gestation
b. 20 to 24 weeks' gestation
c. 28 to 32 weeks' gestation
d. 36 to 40 weeks' gestation

61. A 32-year-old gravida 4, para 2 at 37 weeks' gestation is admitted to the delivery suite with the diagnosis of abruptio placentae. With this complication of pregnancy, blood loss may be:
a. unobserved
b. minimal
c. greater than observed
d. less than observed

62. The nurse notes the physician's orders for the previous client. Which of the following orders will be of highest priority?
a. Type and cross-match for whole blood
b. Assessment of maternal vital signs
c. Assessment of fetal heart rate
d. Measurement of fundal height

63. The main reason for a 3-week restriction on resuming sexual intercourse after birth is to prevent:
a. tearing the episiotomy site
b. vaginal and cervical infection
c. postpartum hemorrhage
d. dyspareunia

64. A 35-year-old woman who has delivered her third child and smokes one pack of cigarettes per day will probably be advised to choose which of the following contraceptive methods?
a. Spermicide
b. Birth control pills
c. Sterilization
d. Intrauterine device

65. A woman using a diaphragm for contraception should be advised to leave it in place against the vagina for how long after intercourse?
a. 1 hour
b. 12 hours
c. 28 hours
d. 6 hours

66. Which of the following situations would warrant remeasurement and possible refitting of a diaphragm?
a. Weight gain of 5 lb
b. Surgery involving general anesthesia
c. Surgery involving regional anesthesia
d. Pregnancy and birth

67. A couple has been unable to conceive during the 5 years of their marriage. They have never used contraception. They report particular pleasure with the use of additional lubrication with petroleum jelly. The man's sperm count is lower than normal, but other assessment data appear to be well within normal limits. Your recommendation for potentially increasing fertility would include which of the following?
a. Have clients reduce frequency of intercourse to less than once a week.
b. Encourage clients to strive for greater consistency in how they perform intercourse.
c. Instruct clients to eliminate the additional lubrication.
d. Clarify the validity of the degree of sexual satisfaction.

68. Introduction of radiopaque material into the uterus and fallopian tubes to assess tubal patency is which of the following diagnostic procedures?
a. Uterotubal insufflation
b. Laparoscopy
c. Culdoscopy
d. Hysterosalpingography

69. About 1 month after delivery, a client comes to the clinic with a fever, hard and inflamed breasts, sore nipples,

and tender axillary lymph nodes. The physician diagnoses mastitis and prescribes treatment. When the client asks you what she should do about breast-feeding her newborn, your best advice to her is:

a. "Stop breast-feeding until your breasts heal."

b. "If possible, try to continue breast-feeding as frequently as possible."

c. "Breast-feed your baby every other day, but first clean your nipples with alcohol."

d. "Breast-feeding during mastitis will cause your milk to dry up."

70. A client admitted to the emergency room following a car accident is in her third trimester of pregnancy. She states she was wearing her seatbelt. She has no external evidence of injury, but she reports extreme abdominal pain. Her abdomen is enlarging and is rigid on palpation. Fetal monitoring indicates acute fetal distress. The client is most likely experiencing which of the following complications?

a. Placenta previa

b. Abruptio placentae

c. Severe abdominal bruising

d. Normal labor stimulated by stress

71. The interventions best suited for the previous client include:

a. monitoring maternal physiologic status

b. monitoring maternal and newborn physiologic status

c. providing emotional support regarding the imminent delivery of a dead or defective newborn

d. administering a tocolytic agent to arrest labor

72. A 25-year-old multigravida is admitted to the hospital in labor. After examining the client, the physician notes on the chart "left anterior face presentation." The landmark used to designate the fetal position in the pelvis is the:

a. acromion

b. mentum

c. occiput

d. sacrum

73. What is the position of the fetal head in a face presentation?

a. Completely flexed

b. Completely extended

c. Partially extended

d. Partially flexed

74. A 22-year-old primigravida is examined in the labor unit. The nurse detects a breech presentation in the left anterior position. Which landmark is used to designate the position in the pelvis of a breech presentation?

a. Acromion

b. Mentum

c. Occiput

d. Sacrum

75. With a left anterior breech presentation, where would the fetal heart rate be most audible?

a. Above the maternal umbilicus and to the left of midline

b. Above the maternal umbilicus and to the right of midline

c. In the lower left maternal abdominal quadrant

d. In the lower right maternal abdominal quadrant

76. At 10:12 AM, the nurse notes that the client's membranes have ruptured, with leakage of greenish fluid. What substance would account for this color?

a. Blood

b. Meconium

c. Hydramnios

d. Caput

77. With a breech presentation, the nurse must be particularly alert for which of the following?

a. Quickening

b. Ophthalmia neonatorum

c. Pica

d. Prolapsed umbilical cord

78. Fetal distress may be indicated by which of the following?

a. Bloody show
b. Hydramnios
c. Oligohydramnios
d. Meconium

79. In the situation outlined in the preceding question, which of the following interventions would receive the highest priority?
   a. Assess fetal heart rate.
   b. Call the physician.
   c. Assess maternal vital signs.
   d. Assess maternal emotional status.

80. A boy is born at 1:10 PM. The Apgar score is taken at 1 minute and again at 5 minutes. Which of the following 1- and 5-minute Apgar scores indicates the newborn is making an appropriate transition to extrauterine life?
   a. 1-minute, 2; 5-minute, 5
   b. 1-minute, 4; 5-minute, 6
   c. 1-minute, 5; 5-minute, 7
   d. 1-minute, 8; 5-minute, 9

81. The newborn can increase body heat by all of the following mechanisms *except*:
   a. crying vigorously
   b. shivering like an adult
   c. metabolizing brown fat
   d. increasing metabolic rate

82. During a physical assessment of a newborn, which of the following comparative measurements would necessitate additional investigation?
   a. Head circumference, 34 cm; chest circumference, 31 cm
   b. Head circumference, 31 cm; chest circumference, 33 cm
   c. Head circumference, 34.5 cm; chest circumference, 32 cm
   d. Head circumference, 32 cm; chest circumference, 30 cm

83. Cold stress is harmful to a newborn because it can lead to which of the following outcomes?
   a. Peripheral vasodilation
   b. Alkalosis
   c. Decreased metabolic activity
   d. Acidosis

84. Nonshivering thermogenesis is a means of increasing body temperature through:
   a. increased muscle activity
   b. metabolism of subcutaneous fat
   c. increased metabolic activity
   d. metabolism of brown fat

85. A newborn weighing 3,000 g and feeding every 4 hours needs 120 calories/kg of body weight every 24 hours for proper growth and development. How many ounces of 20 cal/oz formula should this newborn receive at each feeding to meet nutritional needs?
   a. 2 oz
   b. 3 oz
   c. 4 oz
   d. 6 oz

86. A woman who has acquired immunodeficiency syndrome (AIDS) has just delivered a 4.5-lb preterm newborn. The newborn has a large forehead, oblique eyes, and a flattened nose bridge. Which of the following nursing interventions is an immediate priority for this newborn?
   a. Report the birth of an infected newborn to the Centers for Disease Control and Prevention in Atlanta as part of your accountability and documentation.
   b. Protect the newborn from ineffective thermoregulation and impaired gas exchange.
   c. Support the mother and her partner as they deal with the crisis of the mother and newborn having AIDS.
   d. Monitor the immunoglobulin and serum antibodies to determine severity of infection and antibody reserves.

87. Throughout the world, the leading cause of maternal death is:
   a. puerperal infection
   b. thrombophlebitis
   c. postpartum hemorrhage
   d. uterine inversion

88. Phototherapy has been initiated for a

newborn to treat hyperbilirubinemia. Which of the following nursing interventions would be inappropriate and could cause injury to the newborn?
   a. Placing the nude newborn in the isolette 18 in from the phototherapy light
   b. Turning the newborn every 2 hours
   c. Rubbing an oil-based lotion on newborn's skin to prevent drying and cracking
   d. Covering the newborn's eyes with protective patches

89. A twin born 1 day ago has an undeveloped right hand with a small thumb and forefinger but only little skin flaps for the other three fingers. The mother refuses to discuss the anomaly and will not look at the newborn's hand or ask to hold it. The mother's reaction could be analyzed as which of the following?
   a. A typical grief reaction of denial
   b. An unnaturally strong preference for one twin over the other
   c. An unhealthy avoidance of dealing with the reality of the newborn's pathology
   d. A pathologic psychological reaction that will greatly interfere with bonding

90. Methergine (methylergonovine) 0.2 mg intramuscularly is ordered for a 23-year-old primipara 3 hours postdelivery who is experiencing postpartum bleeding. Potential side effects of the oxytocic drug include which of the following?
   a. Water intoxication
   b. Sudden hypertension
   c. Severe hypoglycemia
   d. Uterine rupture

91. A client is admitted to the postpartum unit with a continuous drip of magnesium sulfate for pregnancy-induced hypertension. Assessment for signs of eclampsia is necessary for at least how many hours postpartum?

   a. 6 hours
   b. 12 hours
   c. 24 hours
   d. 72 hours

92. Within a few minutes of delivery of a 6-lb boy with Apgars of 4 and 10, the mother complains of severe chest pain. Her respirations are shallow, ranging between 24 and 30 per minute. A pulmonary embolism is detected by lung scan. The mother receives heparin sodium intravenous therapy with periodic coagulation studies. Of the following common postpartum medications, which would be contraindicated by the heparin therapy?
   a. docusate sodium (Colace)
   b. bromocriptine (Parlodel)
   c. ibuprofen (Motrin)
   d. acetaminophen (Tylenol)

93. Of the following complex of symptoms, which one would lead the nurse to advise a client to call her physician?
   a. Scant lochia serosa, fatigue, breast tenderness
   b. Scant lochia serosa, fatigue, perianal soreness
   c. Scant lochia rubra, temperature <101°F, uterine tenderness
   d. Scant lochia alba, fatigue, painful hemorrhoids

94. After cesarean delivery, a client complains of vulvar pain in the area of herpes lesions. Which comfort measure would be most advisable for the nurse to implement?
   a. Encourage her to ambulate several times daily.
   b. Suggest she wear tampons rather than maternity pads.
   c. Apply warm, moist compresses to the vulva several times daily.
   d. Administer sitz baths twice daily; change maternity pads frequently.

95. The nurse's first responsibility in the management of postpartum hemorrhage is to do which of the following?

a. Notify the physician before taking any action.
b. Massage the uterus firmly.
c. Take the woman's vital signs.
d. Call for blood type and cross-match and have intravenous equipment ready.

96. Early postpartum hemorrhage is defined as the loss how much blood during the first 24 hours following delivery?
   a. 100 mL
   b. 200 mL
   c. 350 mL
   d. 500 mL

97. The assessment findings for a client with an incompetent cervix should contain which of the following?
   a. Anxiety and fear related to situational low self-esteem
   b. History of one of her sisters-in-law with the same diagnosis
   c. History of repeated, spontaneous second-trimester termination
   d. The need to discuss the importance of cervical rest with no orgasms

98. Which of the following statements is a key concept related to early postpartum hemorrhage?
   a. Excessive blood loss may produce a change in the mother's vital signs.

b. Postpartum hemorrhage is experienced by about 5% of women following birth.
c. Assess the condition of the skin, urinary output, and level of consciousness.
d. Measure and record maternal vital signs after delivery—every 5 to 15 minutes.

99. A positive Homans' sign indicates which of the following?
   a. Possible mastitis
   b. Probable urinary tract infection
   c. Possible postpartum hemorrhage
   d. Probable deep vein thrombosis

100. Identify factors associated with post-maturity in the post-term newborn.
   a. First pregnancies, grand multiparity, history of prolonged pregnancy, anencephaly, and trisomy 16 to 18
   b. History of prolonged pregnancy, pneumothorax, potential hypoglycemia, anencephaly, and trisomy 16 to 18
   c. Meconium aspiration syndrome, grand multiparity, trisomy 16 to 18, parchment-like skin, and Seckel's dwarfism
   d. First pregnancy, Seckel's dwarfism, trisomy 16 to 18, anencephaly, multiparity, and pneumothorax

# Answer Sheet for Comprehensive Exam

*With a pencil, blacken the circle under the option you have chosen for your correct answer.*

| | A | B | C | D | | A | B | C | D | | A | B | C | D |
|---|---|---|---|---|---|---|---|---|---|---|---|---|---|---|
| 1. | ○ | ○ | ○ | ○ | 21. | ○ | ○ | ○ | ○ | 41. | ○ | ○ | ○ | ○ |
| 2. | ○ | ○ | ○ | ○ | 22. | ○ | ○ | ○ | ○ | 42. | ○ | ○ | ○ | ○ |
| 3. | ○ | ○ | ○ | ○ | 23. | ○ | ○ | ○ | ○ | 43. | ○ | ○ | ○ | ○ |
| 4. | ○ | ○ | ○ | ○ | 24. | ○ | ○ | ○ | ○ | 44. | ○ | ○ | ○ | ○ |
| 5. | ○ | ○ | ○ | ○ | 25. | ○ | ○ | ○ | ○ | 45. | ○ | ○ | ○ | ○ |
| 6. | ○ | ○ | ○ | ○ | 26. | ○ | ○ | ○ | ○ | 46. | ○ | ○ | ○ | ○ |
| 7. | ○ | ○ | ○ | ○ | 27. | ○ | ○ | ○ | ○ | 47. | ○ | ○ | ○ | ○ |
| 8. | ○ | ○ | ○ | ○ | 28. | ○ | ○ | ○ | ○ | 48. | ○ | ○ | ○ | ○ |
| 9. | ○ | ○ | ○ | ○ | 29. | ○ | ○ | ○ | ○ | 49. | ○ | ○ | ○ | ○ |
| 10. | ○ | ○ | ○ | ○ | 30. | ○ | ○ | ○ | ○ | 50. | ○ | ○ | ○ | ○ |
| 11. | ○ | ○ | ○ | ○ | 31. | ○ | ○ | ○ | ○ | 51. | ○ | ○ | ○ | ○ |
| 12. | ○ | ○ | ○ | ○ | 32. | ○ | ○ | ○ | ○ | 52. | ○ | ○ | ○ | ○ |
| 13. | ○ | ○ | ○ | ○ | 33. | ○ | ○ | ○ | ○ | 53. | ○ | ○ | ○ | ○ |
| 14. | ○ | ○ | ○ | ○ | 34. | ○ | ○ | ○ | ○ | 54. | ○ | ○ | ○ | ○ |
| 15. | ○ | ○ | ○ | ○ | 35. | ○ | ○ | ○ | ○ | 55. | ○ | ○ | ○ | ○ |
| 16. | ○ | ○ | ○ | ○ | 36. | ○ | ○ | ○ | ○ | 56. | ○ | ○ | ○ | ○ |
| 17. | ○ | ○ | ○ | ○ | 37. | ○ | ○ | ○ | ○ | 57. | ○ | ○ | ○ | ○ |
| 18. | ○ | ○ | ○ | ○ | 38. | ○ | ○ | ○ | ○ | 58. | ○ | ○ | ○ | ○ |
| 19. | ○ | ○ | ○ | ○ | 39. | ○ | ○ | ○ | ○ | 59. | ○ | ○ | ○ | ○ |
| 20. | ○ | ○ | ○ | ○ | 40. | ○ | ○ | ○ | ○ | 60. | ○ | ○ | ○ | ○ |

270

|     | A | B | C | D |
|-----|---|---|---|---|
| 61. | ○ | ○ | ○ | ○ |
| 62. | ○ | ○ | ○ | ○ |
| 63. | ○ | ○ | ○ | ○ |
| 64. | ○ | ○ | ○ | ○ |
| 65. | ○ | ○ | ○ | ○ |
| 66. | ○ | ○ | ○ | ○ |
| 67. | ○ | ○ | ○ | ○ |
| 68. | ○ | ○ | ○ | ○ |
| 69. | ○ | ○ | ○ | ○ |
| 70. | ○ | ○ | ○ | ○ |
| 71. | ○ | ○ | ○ | ○ |
| 72. | ○ | ○ | ○ | ○ |
| 73. | ○ | ○ | ○ | ○ |
| 74. | ○ | ○ | ○ | ○ |

|     | A | B | C | D |
|-----|---|---|---|---|
| 75. | ○ | ○ | ○ | ○ |
| 76. | ○ | ○ | ○ | ○ |
| 77. | ○ | ○ | ○ | ○ |
| 78. | ○ | ○ | ○ | ○ |
| 79. | ○ | ○ | ○ | ○ |
| 80. | ○ | ○ | ○ | ○ |
| 81. | ○ | ○ | ○ | ○ |
| 82. | ○ | ○ | ○ | ○ |
| 83. | ○ | ○ | ○ | ○ |
| 84. | ○ | ○ | ○ | ○ |
| 85. | ○ | ○ | ○ | ○ |
| 86. | ○ | ○ | ○ | ○ |
| 87. | ○ | ○ | ○ | ○ |

|      | A | B | C | D |
|------|---|---|---|---|
| 88.  | ○ | ○ | ○ | ○ |
| 89.  | ○ | ○ | ○ | ○ |
| 90.  | ○ | ○ | ○ | ○ |
| 91.  | ○ | ○ | ○ | ○ |
| 92.  | ○ | ○ | ○ | ○ |
| 93.  | ○ | ○ | ○ | ○ |
| 94.  | ○ | ○ | ○ | ○ |
| 95.  | ○ | ○ | ○ | ○ |
| 96.  | ○ | ○ | ○ | ○ |
| 97.  | ○ | ○ | ○ | ○ |
| 98.  | ○ | ○ | ○ | ○ |
| 99.  | ○ | ○ | ○ | ○ |
| 100. | ○ | ○ | ○ | ○ |

1. **Correct response: a**
   Bartholin's glands are the glands on either side of the vaginal orifice.
   **b.** The clitoris is female erectile tissue.
   **c.** The parotid gland opens into the mouth.
   **d.** Skene's glands open into the posterior wall of the female urinary meatus.
   *Analysis/Physiologic/Analysis (Dx)*

2. **Correct response: b**
   Labia majora are raised longitudinal folds of adipose tissue.
   **a.** Labia minora are soft longitudinal folds of skin between the labia majora.
   **c.** The mons pubis is a mound of fatty tissue over the symphysis pubis.
   **d.** The vestibule is the almond-shaped area between the labia minora.
   *Knowledge/Safe Care/Assessment*

3. **Correct response: d**
   A platypelloid pelvis is a flat female pelvis with a transverse oval inlet.
   **a, b, and c.** These describe a gynecoid pelvis, an android pelvis, and an anthropoid pelvis, respectively.
   *Knowledge/Safe Care/Assessment*

4. **Correct response: c**
   The fundus is the upper rounded portion of the uterus between the fallopian tubes.
   **a.** The corpus is the body of the uterus.
   **b.** The decidua is the mucous lining of the uterus during pregnancy.
   **d.** The isthmus is a uterine structure located above the cervix.
   *Application/Safe Care/Assessment*

5. **Correct response: b**
   The obstetric conjugate should measure 11 cm.

   **a, c, and d.** These are all incorrect answers.
   *Analysis/Physiologic/Assessment*

6. **Correct response: d**
   Secretion of estrogen by the fetal gonad results in differentiation as a girl.
   **a.** Increased maternal estrogen secretion occurs in all pregnancies.
   **b.** Maternal androgen secretion remains the same as before pregnancy.
   **c.** Secretion of androgen by the fetal gonad would differentiate a male fetus.
   *Analysis/Physiologic/Analysis (Dx)*

7. **Correct response: c**
   Gravida refers to a pregnant woman; para refers to a woman who has given birth to a viable infant.
   **a, b, and d.** See the definitions of gravida and para above.
   *Application/Safe Care/NA*

8. **Correct response: a**
   Human chorionic gonadotropin is measured to confirm diagnosis of pregnancy.
   **b.** This is a hormone produced by the ovary.
   **c.** This is a hormone produced by the anterior pituitary in the first half of the menstrual cycle.
   **d.** This is a hormone produced by the corpus luteum and placenta. It stimulates proliferation of the endometrium and growth of the embryo.
   *Knowledge/Safe Care/Assessment*

9. **Correct response: b**
   Presumptive changes suggest but do not confirm pregnancy.
   **a.** This is not considered a categoric change of pregnancy.
   **c.** Probable changes strongly suggest pregnancy.

272

d. Positive changes are diagnostic of pregnancy.
*Comprehension/Safe Care/Assessment*

10. **Correct response: b**
    Chadwick's sign is a blue-purple cervix and vaginal mucous membrane.
    a. Braxton's sign refers to painless intermittent contractions that begin in the fourth month of pregnancy.
    c. Softening of the cervix is Goodell's sign.
    d. Flexibility of the body of the uterus against the cervix is McDonald's sign.
    *Knowledge/Safe Care/Assessment*

11. **Correct response: b**
    This is done to relieve pressure on the vena cava.
    a. This will relieve pressure on vena cava but may exacerbate feelings of faintness.
    c. This will not relieve symptoms; the pressure on the vena cava must be reduced.
    d. Decreasing pressure on the vena cava will cause symptoms to subside.
    *Comprehension/Physiologic/ Implementation*

12. **Correct response: c**
    This will help to reduce the muscle cramps immediately.
    a. This may decrease discomfort but will not reduce the cramp in the muscle.
    b. This may help to relax the muscle in time, but the cramp must be reduced immediately to relieve discomfort.
    d. This will not reduce the cramp in the muscle
    *Comprehension/Physiologic/ Implementation*

13. **Correct response: c**
    Ballottement refers to passive movement of the unengaged fetus.
    a. This is not a contraction but

rather the passive movement of the unengaged fetus.
    b. This refers to quickening.
    d. This is Piskacek's sign.
    *Knowledge/Physiologic/Implementation*

14. **Correct response: d**
    This needs evaluation; it could be an abnormal finding because the upper left outer quadrant is where a great number of cancerous lumps are found.
    **a, b, and c.** These are all normal findings during pregnancy.
    *Analysis/Health Promotion/Evaluation*

15. **Correct response: d**
    Ideally, a woman gains about 1 lb a week during the second and third trimesters.
    a. Usually 2 to 4 lb are gained in the first trimester.
    b. This is not wrong, but it is not as precise as answer d.
    c. A steady weight gain is important for fetal well-being.
    *Application/Safe Care/Implementation*

16. **Correct response: b**
    Ultrasonography can help determine gestational age and the approximate date of delivery.
    a. Determining sex can be incorrect, and ultrasonography is not done for this purpose.
    c. Unfortunately, this is correct; however, it is not advisable to tell clients this.
    d. Later fetal anomalies may be seen, but early fetal anomalies need further testing.
    *Analysis/Safe Care/Implementation*

17. **Correct response: a**
    This is not appropriate because it can increase sodium content.
    b. Regular crackers usually have a high sodium content.
    c. Dry meals often decrease nausea.
    d. Keeping the stomach full often decreases nausea.
    *Analysis/Safe Care/Implementation*

18. **Correct response: b**
    Alcohol consumption during pregnancy is associated with fetal defects; no safe amount of consumption has been established.
    **a, c, and d.** Alcohol should be avoided throughout pregnancy.
*Application/Safe Care/Implementation*

19. **Correct response: c**
    Breathing techniques help raise the pain threshold and reduce the perception of pain.
    **a.** Pain is not eliminated.
    **b.** Position, not breathing, increases uteroplacental perfusion.
    **d.** Breathing techniques can reduce, but not eliminate, pain.
*Analysis/Physiologic/Analysis (Dx)*

20. **Correct response: a**
    Counterpressure eases discomfort.
    **b.** The fetus rotates because of fetal position and configuration of the pelvis.
    **c.** Only midforceps rotation could turn the fetus, and this is not often done.
    **d.** This may contribute to the backache, but it is not the best answer.
*Analysis/Physiologic/Planning*

21. **Correct response: c**
    Arrest of labor is frequent in women with android pelves.
    **a.** This response would be irrelevant to the situation.
    **b.** A platypelloid pelvis, not an android pelvis, is contracted.
    **d.** It is inappropriate to offer false hope. She may have to have a cesarean delivery.
*Analysis/Health Promotion/Planning*

22. **Correct response: d**
    This theory poses that the release of a complex cascade of bioactive agents from the uterine decidua into the amniotic fluid triggers labor.
    **a.** According to this theory, the uterus is increasingly sensitive to oxytocin as pregnancy advances.

    **b.** This theory poses that lipids trigger steroids and release precursors that increase the synthesis of prostaglandin.
    **c.** Proponents of this theory think that progesterone keeps the uterine smooth muscle from contracting throughout pregnancy; near term, the placenta produces less progesterone, which initiates labor.
*Analysis/Physiologic/Assessment*

23. **Correct response: d**
    This condition may lead to a transverse lie.
    **a and b.** These have nothing to do with a transverse lie.
    **c.** The capacity of the uterus is the same for all women unless pathology is present.
*Analysis/Safe Care/Assessment*

24. **Correct response: c**
    Back pain is common in pregnancy and is not a sign of impending labor.
    **a, b, and d.** These are all signs of impending labor.
*Comprehension/Health Promotion/Assessment*

25. **Correct response: a**
    The active phase is when the cervix dilates from about 3 to 10 cm.
    **b.** Stage two begins with complete dilatation of the cervix and ends with delivery of the newborn.
    **c.** Stage three ends with delivery of the placenta.
    **d.** Stage four is 1 to 4 hours after delivery.
*Knowledge/Physiologic/Analysis (Dx)*

26. **Correct response: d**
    The heart rate, respiratory effort, muscle tone, reflex irritability, and color are each given a score of 2.
    **a, b, and c:** All are incorrect responses.
*Analysis/Physiologic/Analysis (Dx)*

**27. Correct response: c**
The newborn must be suctioned and respirations established to maintain life.
**a.** Blankets are not used to cover a newborn in a radiant warmer because the heat warms the outer surface of objects. Also, the newborn's color must be observable.
**b and d.** Although these are important, neither is the first priority.
*Application/Physiologic/Planning*

**28. Correct response: b**
To facilitate drainage of mucus, place the newborn in a lateral position with the head slightly lowered.
**a.** In this position, the newborn lies laterally with the top knee and thigh drawn up toward the chest.
**b.** In this position, the newborn lies supine with the legs and thighs flexed up to the abdomen.
**d.** In this position, the newborn lies supine on a flat surface.
*Application/Physiologic/Planning*

**29. Correct response: a**
A distended bladder will elevate and displace the uterus in the abdomen.
**b.** A displaced uterus is generally an indication of a full bladder. Vigorous massage of the uterus will cause unnecessary discomfort.
**c.** Oxytocic drugs are administered only if the uterus becomes boggy and will not contract.
**d.** Tocolytic drugs are used to relax the uterus and to prevent or stop premature labor.
*Application/Safe Care/Implementation*

**30. Correct response: b**
The nurse's primary responsibility immediately after delivery is to observe for postpartum hemorrhage.
**a.** The fundus should not be massaged vigorously, because this will cause discomfort and may overstimulate the uterus.
**c and d.** These are poor responses, because the nurse offers no explanation of why a procedure is being done.
*Comprehension/Physiologic/Planning*

**31. Correct response: a**
Right after delivery, the fundus should be in the midline midway between the umbilicus and the symphysis pubis.
**b.** This would indicate that the bladder is full.
**c.** This would indicate that the uterus has relaxed and needs gentle massage.
**d.** This indicates that the bladder is full and that the uterus has relaxed.
*Comprehension/Safe Care/Planning*

**32. Correct response: a**
With hypotonic dysfunction, uterine contractions decrease in strength, as does uterine tone. The contractions are not strong enough to produce cervical dilation.
**b.** In hypertonic uterine dysfunction, the uterus does not relax completely between contractions, and contractions are of poor quality.
**c.** Dystocia due to variations in the passageway interferes with engagement, descent, and expulsion of the fetus and can be the cause of hypotonic dysfunction.
**d.** Weak, ineffective contractions cause maternal fatigue; contractions are not affected by maternal state of rest.
*Analysis/Health Promotion/Physiologic*

**33. Correct response: c**
Maternal and fetal vital signs must be monitored closely to determine the physiologic status and well-being of the maternal–fetal unit.
**a.** This is not an indication of hemorrhage at this time.
**b and d.** While important, the priority is to evaluate the integrity of the maternal–fetal unit.

*Analysis/Safe Care/Planning*

**34. Correct response: d**
Oxytocin will augment contractions; therefore, it is essential to evaluate the contractions for frequency, duration, and intensity to prevent overstimulation of the uterus.

**a, b, and c.** These are important to assess, but they are not the highest priority.

*Analysis/Safe Care/Planning*

**35. Correct response: d**
A sterile vaginal examination would not be done because it could cause hemorrhage. Until a diagnosis is made, no vaginal examination is indicated.

**a.** Assessment of maternal vital signs is important to determine maternal physiologic status.

**b.** Assessment of the fetal heart rate (FHR) is essential to determine fetal well-being.

**c.** Assessment of contractions for frequency, duration, and intensity is important when evaluating the progress of labor.

*Analysis/Safe Care/Implementation*

**36. Correct response: d**
The cardinal symptom of placenta previa is painless, bright red vaginal bleeding during the last half of pregnancy.

**a.** The cardinal symptom of abruptio placentae is a painful, boardlike uterus with dark red or no vaginal bleeding.

**b.** Bloody show is a pink mucous discharge after the discharge of the mucous plug. Show is caused by the fetal presenting part pressing against the cervix and rupturing capillaries.

**c.** In ectopic pregnancy, the embryo is implanted in a site other than the uterine cavity.

*Application/Safe Care/Assessment*

**37. Correct response: c**
External monitoring will produce a continuous recording of the FHR and show the fetal response to maternal contractions.

**a.** A clear, accurate FHR cannot always be obtained with a stethoscope.

**b.** FHR is taken periodically with a fetoscope; a continuous recording is preferred to show continuous fetal response.

**d.** An internal monitor is not used during labor, because the placenta is at the internal cervical os.

*Comprehension/Safe Care/Assessment*

**38. Correct response: d**
With cervical dilation and effacement, the placenta will continue to break away from the site of implantation and cause bleeding.

**a, b, and c.** These are important aspects to determine but not of the highest priority.

*Comprehension/Physiologic/Assessment*

**39. Correct response: d**
The nurse should explain what the physician meant by "complete placenta previa" and why the cesarean section is needed.

**a.** This is a poor response that would increase the client's anxiety.

**b.** It is true that a cesarean section would help prevent further hemorrhage, but this statement does not explain the reason for the cesarean delivery.

**c.** In a complete placenta previa, the total internal cervical os is covered by the placenta.

*Application/Safe Care/Implementation*

**40. Correct response: a**
The placenta is low or covering the cervical os and fetus and may not allow for vertical position.

**b.** This is separation of a normally implanted placenta.

**c and d.** These are examples of normal attachment.
*Analysis/Physiologic/Analysis (Dx)*

**41. Correct response: c**
Radiographic pelvimetry will give the most accurate measurement.
**a.** This will show soft tissue.
**b.** This is not done without further evaluation.
**d.** This is not as accurate as pelvimetry and generally is not done during labor.
*Analysis/Safe Care/Evaluation*

**42. Correct response: b**
At 14 to 16 weeks, the uterus is sufficiently out of the pelvis to remove the needed fluid. Also, the pregnancy is sufficiently early to terminate in the event of a fetal defect.
**a.** At 8 to 10 weeks' gestation, amniocentesis is considered risky.
**c and d.** After 26 weeks' gestation, termination of pregnancy because of fetal defect is not recommended.
*Knowledge/Health Promotion/ Assessment*

**43. Correct response: d**
Typically, infants of diabetic mothers (IDM) are large for gestational age, less mature, and at increased risk for respiratory distress and tremors associated with hypoglycemia.
**a.** Jaundice, hydrocephalus, and seizures are abnormal in any newborn.
**b.** Because of immaturity, the large IDM could have difficulty maintaining body temperature, but he or she would not necessarily have an enlarged brain.
**c.** Congenital anomalies are common, but hemangiomas or mongolian spots are not.
*Knowledge/Health Promotion/Planning*

**44. Correct response: a**
Urine estriol levels usually rise as pregnancy progresses. Falling levels

suggest some interference with fetal well-being.
**b, c, and d.** These all indicate normal fetal maturity.
*Analysis/Safe Care/Analysis (Dx)*

**45. Correct response: d**
The same circulatory disorders that affect the small blood vessels of the diabetic client also affect the vessels of the placenta, resulting in placental insufficiency and leading to fetal distress.
**a.** Concurrent infections may increase vulnerability in the term diabetic client, but the decision to induce labor depends on additional data.
**b.** Although diabetic mothers tend to have large babies and the incidence of cephalopelvic disproportion is greater for these mothers, the decision to induce labor is based on other factors.
**c.** Although true for some, this is not the basis for determining appropriate birth time.
*Analysis/Safe Care/Planning*

**46. Correct response: b**
These measures are essential for preventing direct transmission of the virus to the newborn.
**a.** The fundus should not be massaged after cesarean delivery.
**c.** This is not necessary and could lead to thrombophlebitis.
**d.** Although it would be helpful to have help with household chores, the mother needs to feel free to mother her newborn to promote attachment.
*Analysis/Safe Care/Planning*

**47. Correct response: a**
Postpartum clients should be instructed to increase fluid intake to prevent this.
**b.** Breast engorgement does not cause elevated temperature in the first 24 hours after delivery.

c. Vaginal infections are rare unless the woman was prone to them before delivery.

d. Uterine infection usually does not occur within 24 hours of delivery.

*Analysis/Physiologic/Analysis (Dx)*

48. *Correct response: a*

This is an infection of the uterine lining.

b. This is a complicated endocrine problem that can cause gynecologic and infertility problems.

c. This is infection of the tube and may occur if endometritis is not cured.

d. This is clot formation in pelvic vessels.

*Analysis/Physiologic/Planning*

49. *Correct response: a*

The birth of twins and long labor could weaken, tire, and overstretch the uterine muscles, making postpartum hemorrhage possible.

b, c, and d. All are incorrect.

*Analysis/Safe Care/Planning*

50. *Correct response: c*

This is the best answer because the woman does not want to care for her newborn.

a. This is normal behavior; many women are exhilarated.

b. Due to hormone changes, this is common.

d. This may be because of anxiety or lack of knowledge.

*Analysis/Psychosocial/Planning*

51. *Correct response: c*

This indicates a postpartum hemorrhage.

a and b. These are within normal limits.

d. This is normal after delivery, because the pregnant woman who normally holds fluids rids herself of excess fluids.

*Analysis/Safe Care/Implementation*

52. *Correct response: a*

This is the first thing to assess.

b. If the uterus is firm, massage is not necessary.

c. Retained placenta fragments cause increased bleeding.

d. The uterus may feel soft.

*Analysis/Safe Care/Analysis (Dx)*

53. *Correct response: d*

Infants born to narcotic-addicted mothers have an increase in reflex irritability and often have continuous body movement.

a. They are poor feeders.

b. They have tremors.

c. They have a high-pitched cry.

*Analysis/Safe Care/Analysis (Dx)*

54. *Correct response: c*

They often are smaller.

a. They do not have a larger head.

b. They are not necessarily shorter in length.

d. This is not necessarily true.

*Analysis/Physiologic/Analysis (Dx)*

55. *Correct response: b*

Bilirubin needs to be monitored.

a. This is too early for physiologic jaundice.

c. Breast-fed babies do have more jaundice, but this is too early for physiologic jaundice.

d. The parents should not be frightened unnecessarily.

*Analysis/Safe Care/Analysis (Dx)*

56. *Correct response: c*

Anemia limits the amount of oxygen available in the body.

a. Extreme tiredness and dizziness are not normal signs of pregnancy.

b. Hemoglobin and hematocrit reflect anemia.

d. Subjective and objective data do not support development of preeclampsia.

*Analysis/Physiologic/Analysis (Dx)*

**57. *Correct response: d***
There is an increased incidence of premature labor and delivery.
a. Infants are often larger due to fetal hyperinsulinism and hyperglycemia.
b. Diabetes is not demonstrated in the fetus or newborn.
c. This type of response will cause more apprehension in the woman.
*Comprehension/Psychosocial/Implementation*

**58. *Correct response: d***
Typically, because of progressive insulin resistance, the client may require a dosage adjustment during pregnancy. The decision will be based on the client's blood glucose levels.
a. This will not help answer the client's question nor solve her problem. The nurse should help her or note her concern.
b. This response may confuse or frighten the client.
c. As above, these answers may cause the client increased anxiety.
*Analysis/Psychosocial/Implemention*

**59. *Correct response: b***
A frequent cough is a primary sign of congestive heart failure.
a. This is a probable change of pregnancy.
c. This is a presumptive change of pregnancy.
d. This is produced by the mammary gland during pregnancy before the onset of lactation.
*Application/Health Promotion/Evaluation*

**60. *Correct response: c***
Progressive rise in cardiac output reaches its peak at 28 to 32 weeks' gestation because there is a peak increase in blood volume, stroke volume, and heart rate at this time.
a, b, and d. These time frames are incorrect.

*Comprehension/Physiologic/Implementation*

**61. *Correct response: c***
With abruptio placentae, there may be concealed hemorrhage with blood loss greater than that observed.
a and b. There is blood loss with abruptio placentae because the placenta tears from the uterus and causes bleeding.
d. Concealed hemorrhage produces *more* blood loss than can be observed.
*Comprehension/Physiologic/Assessment*

**62. *Correct response: a***
Blood loss can be great; therefore, blood replacement is the highest priority.
b, c, and d. These are important but not the highest priority.
*Comprehension/Health promotion/Planning*

**63. *Correct response: b***
A woman is at increased risk for vaginal and cervical infection for the first 3 weeks after delivery.
a. The episiotomy is usually fairly well healed in the first week.
c. This statement is not true.
d. This may be true, but it is not the best answer.
*Analysis/Physiologic/Planning*

**64. *Correct response: d***
Of those mentioned, it is the most effective except for sterilization, a largely irreversible method of contraception.
a. Spermicide is less convenient and less effective than an intrauterine device.
b. Oral contraceptives are not given to older women who smoke because of the possibility of embolism problems.
c. Sterilization would not be recommended because of its permanency.
*Analysis/Safe Care/Planning*

**65. Correct response: d**
The diaphragm should remain in place at least 6 hours after each (if applicable) subsequent intercourse.
**a, b, and c.** These are incorrect responses.
*Analysis/Safe Care/Implementation*

**66. Correct response: d**
This can change the shape or size of pelvic structures, and refitting of the diaphragm may be necessary.
**a.** A weight gain or loss of 15 lb or more is the benchmark indicating that refitting may be necessary.
**b and c.** Anesthesia does not have anything to do with anatomic changes of the pelvis.
*Analysis/Health Promotion/
Implementation*

**67. Correct response: c**
Petroleum jelly and some water-soluble lubricants have been shown to be spermicidal.
**a.** Reducing intercourse will not increase the probability of conception.
**b and d.** The data at this point do not support these as factors in this couple's inability to conceive.
*Analysis/Safe Care/Implementation*

**68. Correct response: d**
Hysterosalpingography involves radiologic examination of the uterine cavity, fallopian tubes, and peritubal area.
**a, b, and c.** These procedures do not use a radiopaque material.

**69. Correct response: b**
Breast-feeding despite mastitis will prevent stasis of the milk glands and thereby promote healing.
**a.** If the mother stops breast-feeding, the milk flow may subside permanently.
**c.** This is poor advice, and cleaning the breasts with alcohol will cause drying and cracking.
**d.** Breast-feeding during mastitis promotes continuing milk flow.
*Application/Health Promotion/Planning*

**70. Correct response: b**
These assessment data point to abruptio placentae.
**a, c, and d.** The assessment data are typical of abruptio placentae and do not support any of the other disorders listed.
*Application/Physiologic/Analysis (Dx)*

**71. Correct response: b**
Both mother and newborn should be monitored carefully to promote survival and to decrease risk of morbidity.
**a.** The newborn and the mother should be monitored.
**c.** The death or defectiveness of the newborn would probably not be a main focus of action unless the newborn dies or has a morbid condition.
**d.** Tocolytics are contraindicated in abruptio placentae.
*Application/Safe Care/Implementation*

**72. Correct response: b**
The mentum is used as the landmark to determine fetal position in a face presentation.
**a.** The acromion is the landmark used for a shoulder presentation.
**c.** The occiput is the landmark used for a vertex presentation.
**d.** The sacrum is the landmark used for a breech presentation.
*Comprehension/Physiology/Assessment*

**73. Correct response: b**
With a face presentation, the head is completely extended.
**a.** The head is completely flexed in a vertex presentation.
**c and d.** Partial extension or flexion can occur in other presentations.
*Comprehension/Safe Care/Assessment*

**74. Correct response: d**
The sacrum is used as the landmark to designate the position of a breech presentation in the pelvis.
**a.** In a shoulder presentation, the

acromion process (scapula) is used as the landmark.

   **b.** The mentum (chin) is the landmark to designate the position of a face presentation.

   **c.** The occiput is used as the landmark in a vertex presentation.

*Comprehension/Physiologic/Assessment*

**75.** *Correct response: a*
The fetal heart is best heard from the fetal upper torso and through the fetal back. With the left sacral anterior presentation, the fetal upper torso and back face the left upper maternal abdominal wall.

   **b, c, and d.** These locations are not the best spots to ausculatate the fetal heart.

*Application/Health Promotion/*
*Analysis (Dx)*

**76.** *Correct response: b*
With descent into the pelvis, the fetus in a breech presentation will pass meconium due to compression on the intestinal tract.

   **a.** Greenish amniotic fluid is not an indication of bleeding.

   **c.** Hydramnios refers to an excessive amount of amniotic fluid.

   **d.** Caput is the occiput of the fetal head that is at the vaginal introitus just before delivery of the head.

*Analysis/Health Promotion/*
*Analysis (Dx)*

**77.** *Correct response: d*
Space is available between the presenting part and the cervix, through which the cord can slip.

   **a.** Quickening is the woman's first perception of fetal movements.

   **b.** Conjunctivitis in the newborn generally results from maternal gonorrhea.

   **c.** Pica refers to oral intake of nonfood substances, such as cornstarch, dirt, clay, or plaster by a malnourished person, often seen in a child or pregnant woman in

need of nutrients to support growth.

*Analysis/Safe Care/Analysis (Dx)*

**78.** *Correct response: d*
With fetal distress, there is an increase in the peristaltic movement of the intestines; thus, the fetus may expel meconium.

   **a.** Bloody show is the pink mucous discharge that is present after discharge of the mucous plug. Show is caused by pressure from the fetal presenting part on the cervix, causing rupture of capillaries.

   **b.** Hydramnios is an excessive amount of amniotic fluid.

   **c.** Oligohydramnios is a decreased amount of amniotic fluid, frequently seen with a fetal urinary tract anomaly.

*Application/Safe Care/Assessment*

**79.** *Correct response: a*
Meconium-stained amniotic fluid is a sign of fetal distress, and the FHR must be assessed immediately.

   **b, c, and d.** These are important interventions but not the highest priority because of the risk to the fetus.

*Analysis/Health Promotion/Planning*

**80.** *Correct response: d*
Apgar scores between 7 and 9 indicate appropriate initial adjustment of the newborn when the heart rate, respiratory effort, muscle tone, reflex irritability, and color are evaluated.

   **a, b, and c.** These scores indicate a compromised newborn; scores below 4 indicate the newborn is severely depressed.

*Analysis/Safe Care/Assessment*

**81.** *Correct response: b*
Newborns cannot shiver.

   **a, c, and d.** Newborns can raise body heat by crying vigorously, metabolizing brown fat, and increasing metabolic rate.

*Analysis/Physiologic/Evaluation*

**82. *Correct response: b***
The head circumference in a normal newborn is larger than the chest circumference.
**a, c, and d.** These measurements fall within normal limits (the head circumferences are larger than the chest circumferences) and need no further investigation.
*Analysis/Safe Care/Analysis (Dx)*

**83. *Correct response: d***
Cold stress constricts pulmonary vessels and decreases blood flow, causing hypoxia and an increase in ketone bodies. It also increases metabolic rate and, with hypoxia, causes anaerobic glycolysis and metabolic acidosis.
**a.** This is a normal occurrence when the newborn is cold.
**b.** This is the opposite of acidosis.
**c.** Cold stress increases metabolic activity.
*Analysis/Physiologic/Analysis (Dx)*

**84. *Correct response: d***
Cold stress stimulates the sympathetic nervous system to release norepinephrine, which causes the metabolism of brown fat.
**a.** This occurs with vigorous crying.
**b.** This does not occur in newborns.
**c.** This occurs in cold stress of the newborn.
*Analysis/Physiologic/Analysis (Dx)*

**85. *Correct response: b***
Mathematical calculations: 1) 3 kg × 120 calories/kg per day = 360 calories/day; 2) 360 calories/day = six feedings per day = 60 calories per feeding; 3) 360 calories per feeding = 20 calories/oz = 3 oz per feeding.
**a, c, and d.** Based on the calculation, these amounts are incorrect.
*Analysis/Health Promotion/Planning*

**86. *Correct response: b***
Monitoring for and correcting ineffective thermoregulation and impaired gas exchange would be the highest priority for this newborn.

**a, c, and d.** Adequate reporting and documentation, parental support, and determination of infection and antibody levels are important, but newborn thermoregulation and gaseous exchange are priorities.
*Application/Safe Care/Planning*

**87. *Correct response: c***
Up to the present time, uterine hemorrhage was the leading cause of maternal death.
**a.** Puerperal infection occurs in up to 8% of new mothers (the percentage is higher in women who had cesarean delivery), but hemorrhage causes more deaths.
**b.** Thrombophlebitis may lead to life-threatening pulmonary embolism, which is rarer than postpartum hemorrhage.
**d.** Unless corrected, uterine inversion, in which the uterus turns inside out, may be the cause of extreme blood loss and hypovolemic shock.
*Knowledge/Safe Care/Assessment*

**88. *Correct response: c***
Oil-based lotions or ointments should not be used, because they may cause burns when used with phototherapy.
**a, b, and d.** These are correct interventions.
*Application/Safe Care/Implementation*

**89. *Correct response: a***
The inability to discuss or look at the pathology soon after its occurrence is common denial and avoidance that are part of grieving. The mother will need time and nonjudgmental support to deal with her disappointment, sadness, and anger about the newborn's anomaly.
**b, c, and d.** The woman's response is neither unnatural, unhealthy, nor pathologic at this time.
*Analysis/Psychosocial/Analysis (Dx)*

**90.** *Correct response: b*

Hypertension is a potential side effect of methylergonomine.

**a, c, and d.** Water intoxication, severe hypoglycemia, and uterine rupture are not potential side effects of this drug.

*Knowledge/Safe Care/Planning*

**91.** *Correct response: d*

Eclampsia is a possibility for as long as 72 hours after delivery in the client with pregnancy-induced hypertension serious enough to be treated with magnesium sulfate.

**a, b, and c.** Assessment should be maintained for at least 48 hours postpartum.

*Comprehension/Safe Care/Application*

**92.** *Correct response: c*

Ibuprofen is contraindicated in clients receiving heparin therapy because it increases the risk of bleeding.

**a, b, and d.** Docusate sodium (Colace), bromocriptine (Parlodel), and acetaminophen (Tylenol) are all considered compatible with heparin.

*Analysis/Safe Care/Implementation*

**93.** *Correct response: c*

These symptoms suggest postpartum infection and should be explored further.

**a, b, and d.** These are all normal concerns 6 days following delivery.

*Application/Safe Care/Assessment*

**94.** *Correct response: d*

Sitz baths are comforting, and frequent pad changes will help the lesions to dry.

**a.** Ambulation will increase discomfort.

**b.** Newly delivered clients should not be encouraged to wear tampons because of the risk of infection.

**c.** This will keep the lesions moist, and keeping them dry promotes healing.

*Comprehension/Physiologic/Planning*

**95.** *Correct response: b*

The primary cause of postpartum hemorrhage is uterine atony. Fundal massage promotes the contraction of the uterus.

**a.** Notifying the physician is not necessary before independent nursing interventions.

**c and d.** Vital sign monitoring, blood typing, and cross-matching may become necessary, but uterine massage is the initial recommended intervention.

*Knowledge/Safe Care/Implementation*

**96.** *Correct response: c*

By definition, blood loss of 500 mL or more during the first 24 hours following delivery is considered early postpartum hemorrhage.

**a, b, and d.** These amounts do not constitute the definition of early postpartum hemorrhage.

*Knowledge/Physiologic/Assessment*

**97.** *Correct response: c*

The assessment findings would contain a history of repeated, spontaneous second-trimester termination.

**a.** Anxiety, fear, and low self-esteem may occur throughout any pregnancy.

**b.** There is no reason why she should have the same problem as a sister-in-law. There is no direct blood or gene line between them.

**d.** This should be a nursing intervention.

*Analysis/Physiologic/Assessment*

**98.** *Correct response: b*

About 5% of women have some type of postpartum hemorrhage.

**a.** Blood loss may cause a change in the maternal vital signs, but it is only part of the situation.

**c.** Assessing the skin condition, urine output, and level of consciousness are nursing responsibilities for any client.

**d.** This is part of routine nursing care.

*Comprehension/Safe Care/NA*

**99.** *Correct response: d*

The positive Homans' sign (pain in the calf on passive dorsiflexion of the foot) indicates deep vein thrombosis.

**a, b, and c.** All are incorrect responses.

*Application/Physiologic/Analysis (Dx)*

**100.** *Correct response: a*

Some factors associated with postmaturity include first pregnancies, grand multiparity, history of prolonged pregnancy, anencephaly, trisomy 16 to 18, and Seckel's dwarfism.

**b, c, and d.** All are missing important factors or have inappropriate etiologies.

*Analysis/Physiologic/Planning*

# Index

Page numbers followed by *f* indicate figures; those followed by *t* indicate tables.

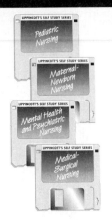
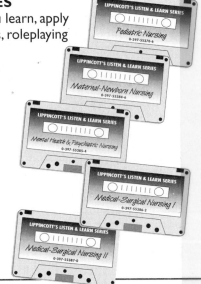
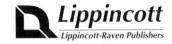